Standard Operating Procedure for Carbon Ion Radiotherapy

碳离子放射治疗
标准操作流程

叶延程　祁　英　主编

编委（按姓氏笔画排序）

马霄云　王开平　卢小丽　孙洁仁　朱芳芳
李万国　李文琪　李菊琴　张一贺　陈东基
陈　喆　杨晓东　孟　莉　孟万斌　段云龙
柴山晃一　康凯丽　鲁会祥

蘭州大學出版社
LANZHOU UNIVERSITY PRESS

图书在版编目（CIP）数据

碳离子放射治疗标准操作流程 / 叶延程，祁英主编
. -- 兰州 : 兰州大学出版社，2018.10
ISBN 978-7-311-05473-1

Ⅰ. ①碳… Ⅱ. ①叶… ②祁… Ⅲ. ①放射治疗学－技术操作规程 Ⅳ. ①R815-65

中国版本图书馆CIP数据核字(2018)第245675号

责任编辑　郝可伟
封面设计　郇　海

书　　名　碳离子放射治疗标准操作流程
作　　者　叶延程　祁　英　主编
出版发行　兰州大学出版社　（地址:兰州市天水南路222号　730000）
电　　话　0931-8912613(总编办公室)　0931-8617156(营销中心)
　　　　　0931-8914298(读者服务部)
网　　址　http://press.lzu.edu.cn
电子信箱　press@lzu.edu.cn
印　　刷　甘肃春宇印务有限公司
开　　本　787 mm×1092 mm　1/16
印　　张　10.75
字　　数　259千
版　　次　2018年10月第1版
印　　次　2018年10月第1次印刷
书　　号　ISBN 978-7-311-05473-1
定　　价　98.00元

前 言

碳离子放射治疗技术是运用碳离子射线对肿瘤区域进行照射从而杀灭肿瘤细胞的治疗技术，是目前国际上最先进的肿瘤放射治疗技术。碳离子射线进入人体后可产生“定向爆破”的效果，使患者得到可喜的疗效。

放射治疗是治疗恶性肿瘤的重要手段，其根本目的是最大限度地消灭肿瘤，同时最大限度地保护正常组织和器官的结构与功能，提高患者的长期生存率和改善其生存质量。碳离子放射治疗技术因其射线进入人体后存在“bragg峰”，相较常规X射线放射治疗技术能更好地控制放射剂量在人体内的分布，可实现对病灶更加精准的治疗，从而在保证靶区剂量足够的情况下最大限度地保护正常组织。

碳离子放射治疗的计划和实施是一个多环节、多步骤的复杂过程，每一个环节之间连接紧密，任一差错都会导致治疗失败。制定此《碳离子治疗标准操作流程》的目的是按规范进行操作，做到质量控制、质量保证。流程中涉及相关专业医务人员的培训和训练、不同放射治疗技术的不断改进、所用设备和辅助器材的操作标准等。此流程可使操作者明晰影响放射治疗质量的关键性因素，从而帮助相关人员更好地按规程操作，使碳离子放射治疗的优点得到最大限度的发挥。

每个人体部位接受总的辐射量是有限度的，以合适的、尽可能高的剂量尽可能精准地照射肿瘤部位，并尽可能减少对周围正常组织的损伤是整个放射治疗过程的根本目标。这不仅需要受过良好专业训练、拥有丰富的治疗经验的医生和物理师、技师团队紧密地团结合作，而且需要在放射治疗过程每一步的操作中做到精准与规范。若操作中出现问题，则可能造成严重后果，如放射治疗后肿瘤因未达到预期照射剂量很快复发、转移，或因放射线对正常组织的损伤导致放射性肺炎、肠穿孔等严重副作用。

由于碳离子放射治疗的高精准性，对患者病灶的照射精确度成为影响放射治疗质量的最大因素。要让射线准确地照射肿瘤病灶，需要做很多的努力，其中很重要的一项是对患者的身体做准确的固定。固定的材料包括可塑形的由特殊材料制作的铺在病人身体下面的真空垫和覆盖在体表的热塑体膜等。固定病人的原则是精度高、重复性好、病人的舒适度好。同时由于患者呼吸运动对肿瘤病灶位置的影响较大，还需采取如图像引导追踪肿瘤、对患者的呼吸运动进行干预等方法提高放射线照射位置的精确性。

制作《碳离子治疗标准操作流程》，旨在提供一些可作为参考的方法，作为碳离子治疗操作的使用助手，为碳离子治疗的规范化做一些尝试。但此项工作只是刚开始，还需在以后的工作中不断摸索、积累经验，进一步改进完善。书中如有不妥之处敬请各位专家、教授批评指正，提出宝贵的意见和建议，以便修订完善。

编者

2018年7月

目 录

第1节 重离子治疗装置物理、技术方面质量保证系统指导方针

Guidelines of Physical and Technological Quality Assurance for Heavy Ion Therapy Devices

………………… 柴山晃一 叶延程 祁英 孟万斌 马霄云 李文琪 001

第2节 trUpoint ARCH用户手册

User Manual of trUpoint ARCH

……………………………… 李万国 张一贺 祁英 孟万斌 马霄云 030

第3节 头颈部肿瘤患者体位固定标准操作流程

Standard Operating Procedure for the Immobilization of Head and Neck Tumor Patients

……………………………… 李万国 张一贺 祁英 孟万斌 马霄云 047

第4节 头颈部肿瘤碳离子放射治疗摆位标准操作流程

Standard Operating Procedure for Carbon Ion Radiotherapy Positioning of Head and Neck Tumor

……………………………… 李文祺 陈东基 祁英 孟万斌 马霄云 052

第5节 胸部肿瘤患者碳离子放射治疗体位固定标准操作流程

Standard Operation Procedure for the Carbon Ion Radiotherapy Immobilization of Chest Tumor Patients

……………………………… 李文祺 陈东基 祁英 孟万斌 马霄云 058

第6节 胸、腹部肿瘤碳离子放射治疗摆位标准操作流程

Standard Operation Procedure for Carbon Ion Radiotherapy of Positioning of Chest and Abdomen Tumor

………………………………………… 鲁会祥 祁英 孟万斌 马霄云 067

第7节 腹部、盆腔肿瘤碳离子放射治疗体位固定标准操作流程

Standard Operation Procedure for Carbon Ion Radiotherapy Treatment

Immobilization of Abdomen and Chest Tumor Patient
……………………………………… 鲁会祥 祁英 孟万斌 马霄云 073

第8节 碳离子放射治疗CT定位标准操作流程
Standard Operating Procedure for CT Localization in Carbon Ion Radiotherapy
……………………………………… 杨晓东 祁英 孟万斌 马霄云 078

第9节 碳离子放射治疗CT机质量保证和质量控制标准操作流程
Standard Operating Procedure for the QA and QC for CT Device in Carbon ion Radiotherapy
……………………………………………………………………… 康凯丽 092

第10节 碳离子放射治疗模拟定位激光灯标准操作流程
Standard Operating Procedure for Carbon Ion Radiotherapy Laser Light
……………………………………… 杨晓东 祁英 孟万斌 马霄云 096

第11节 碳离子放射治疗恒温水箱标准操作流程
Standard Operating Procedure for Carbon Ion Rodiotherapy of Thermostatic Water Tank
…………………………………… 孟莉 孙洁仁 祁英 孟万斌 马霄云 099

第12节 碳离子放射治疗患者转移至治疗室标准操作流程
Standard Operating Procedure for Transporting Patients to the Treatment Room in Carbon Ion Radiotherapy
………………………………… 李文祺 陈东基 祁英 孟万斌 马霄云 102

第13节 碳离子放射治疗真空负压袋体位固定标准操作流程
Standard Operating Procedure for Vacuum Negative Pressure Bag Immobilization of Carbon Ion Radiotherapy
…………………………………… 孟莉 孙洁仁 祁英 孟万斌 马霄云 105

第14节 碳离子放射治疗真空泵标准操作流程
Standard Operating Procedure for Vacuum Pump in Carbon Ion Radiotherapy
……………………………………… 鲁会祥 祁英 孟万斌 马霄云 109

第15节 碳离子放射治疗患者位置确认标准操作流程
Standard Operating Procedure for Patient's Position Verification in Carbon Ion Radiotherapy
……………………………………… 朱芳芳 祁英 孟万斌 马霄云 113

第16节 碳离子放射治疗患者准备间标准操作流程
Standard Operating Procedures for Patients Preparation Room in Carbon Ion Radiotherapy
……………………………………… 朱芳芳 祁英 孟万斌 马霄云 122

第17节　碳离子放射治疗转运床标准操作流程
Standard Operating Procedure for Carbon Ion Therapy Trolley
…………………………………………… 王开平　祁英　孟万斌　马霄云　125
第18节　碳离子计划（ciPlan）设计标准操作流程
Standard Operating Procedure for Carbon Ion Plan Design
…………………………………………… 卢小丽　祁英　孟万斌　马霄云　128
第19节　碳离子放射治疗患者信息导入ciPlan标准操作流程
Standard Operating Procedure for Carbon Ion Radiotherapy Patient Information Importing ciPlan
…………………………………………… 卢小丽　祁英　孟万斌　马霄云　133
第20节　碳离子放射治疗患者信息确认标准操作流程
Standard Operating Procedure for Confirm the Patient's Basic Information for Carbon Ion Radiotherapy
…………………………………………… 段云龙　祁英　孟万斌　马霄云　136
第21节　盆腔、下腹部肿瘤碳离子放射治疗摆位标准操作流程
Standard Operating Procedure for the Position Setting in Carbon Ion Radiotherapy of Pelvic and Lower Abdominal Tumors
…………………………………………… 段云龙　祁英　孟万斌　马霄云　138
第22节　腿部肿瘤碳离子放射治疗摆位标准操作流程
Standard Operating Procedure for Position Setting in Heavy Ion Radiotherapy of Leg Tumors
…………………………………………… 段云龙　祁英　孟万斌　马霄云　141
第23节　手部肿瘤碳离子放射治疗摆位标准操作流程
Standard Operating Procedure for the Position Setting in Carbon Ion Beam Radiotherapy of Arm Tumors
…………………………………………… 段云龙　祁英　孟万斌　马霄云　144
第24节　其他部位肿瘤碳离子放射治疗摆位标准操作流程
Standard Operating Procedure for Position Setting in Carbon Ion Radiotherapy of Other Parts Tumors
…………………………………………… 段云龙　祁英　孟万斌　马霄云　147
第25节　碳离子放射治疗患者转运出治疗室及下床标准操作流程
Standard Operating Procedure for Patients Transfering from the Treatment Room and Getting off Bed in Carbon Ion Rodiotherapy
…………………………………………… 王开平　祁英　孟万斌　马霄云　149

第26节 碳离子放射治疗四肢肿瘤及其他部位肿瘤体位固定标准操作流程
Standard Operating Procedure for Immobilization in Carbon Ion Radiotherapy of Limbs and Other Parts Tumors
…………………………………… 王开平 祁英 孟万斌 马霄云 151
第27节 碳离子放射治疗计划命名标准操作流程
Standard Operating Procedure for Carbon Ion Radiotherapy Plan Naming
…………………………………… 马霄云 祁英 孟万斌 马霄云 154
第28节 高压注射器标准操作流程
Standard Operating Procedure for High Pressure Syringe
……………………………… 陈喆 李菊琴 祁英 孟万斌 马霄云 158
第29节 甘肃重离子医院重离子放射治疗楼辐射事故应急预案
Emergency Plan for Radiation Accidents in Heavy Ion Radiotherapy Buildings of Gansu Heavy Ion Hospital ……………………………………162
参考文献 …………………………………………………………… 178

第1节　重离子治疗装置物理、技术方面质量保证系统指导方针

Guidelines of Physical and Technological Quality Assurance for Heavy Ion Therapy Devices

作者：柴山晃一　叶延程　祁英　孟万斌　马霄云　李文琪

1　保证重离子线治疗精度的项目

(Projects for ensuring the accuracy of heavy ion beam treatment)

从重离子治疗装置的性能考虑，我们应该意识到存在许多与绝对剂量的设定相关的因素。剂量的不确定性不是偶然的误差，而是和系统误差的很多情况有关。这些误差，只要不能明确判断是系统误差，就要作为偶然误差对待。查明系统误差产生的原因，并努力将其从系统中排除，在质量保证工作中是非常重要的。

According to the performance of heavy ion therapy devices, we should be aware that there are many factors associated with setting absolute dose. Dosimetry uncertainty is not an accidental error, but rather a concern with many cases of systematic error. These errors, as long as they can not be clearly judged to be systematic errors, should be treated as accidental errors. Identifying the causes of systematic errors and trying to eliminate them from the system is very important in QA work.

2　基准条件的形成

(Formation of the benchmark conditions)

重离子治疗装置的评价标准，就是单纯化的标准条件照射而形成的剂量分布的精度。测定剂量分布定义质量保证的参数，检查剂量重复性等。

The evaluation criteria for heavy ion therapy devices are the accuracy of the dose distribution formed by simple standard irradiation. Evaluate parameters defined QA by dose distribution and check dose repeatability and others.

3　剂量仪的校对

(Calibration of dosimeter)

通过对患者剂量校对点的剂量测定，来确定每个患者的监控计数（*MU*值）。在计

算放射治疗的*MU*值时，确保剂量标定的准确度是非常必要的。因为每天标定都要使用剂量仪，所以剂量仪的管理非常重要。日常使用的剂量仪有射野剂量仪和参考剂量仪。通常的剂量测定使用射野剂量仪，将它和参考剂量仪进行相互校对。测定剂量时使用的温度计和气压计，要遵从各自的说明书进行定期校对。

Decide monitoring dose（*MU* value）of each patient by measuring dose at the patient dose proofing point. It is necessary to ensure the accuracy of dose calibration when calculating the *MU* value for the radiotherapy. Because dosimeters are used for calibration every day, dosimeter management is very important. Dosimeters for daily use include field dosimeters and reference dosimeters. The usual dosimetry uses a field dosimeter, and it's calibrated with a reference dosimeter. Thermometers and barometers for determining dose should be regularly calibrated in accordance with the respective instructions.

4 参考剂量仪的校对

（Calibration of reference dosimeter）

在重离子治疗开始之前，应该和其他重离子治疗设备剂量进行对比。对比使用的参考剂量仪的灵敏度校对要依据相关规定进行。

We should compare doses with other heavy ion therapy devices before heavy ion therapy. The calibration of the sensitivity of the reference dosimeter should be based on the relevant regulations.

5 射野剂量仪的校对

（Calibration of field dosimeter）

对于X射线、^{60}Co伽马线及离子线使用的剂量仪，至少每半年将其对照参考剂量仪进行校对一次。因为每天的使用会导致剂量仪的灵敏度降低，所以必须进行恰当的精度管理。

For dosimeters used for X-rays, ^{60}Co gamma rays and ion beams, their reference dosimetry should be calibrated at least half year. Because daily use can cause the dosimeter's sensitivity decrease, proper accuracy management must be done.

6 剂量监控系统

（Dose monitoring system）

剂量监控系统是由独立的两个监控剂量和监视照射野的平坦度的系统校对的。独立的束流截断信号从两个剂量监控输出，需要直接地、严格地连接各自的束流开关。治疗束流以脉冲形式发出。在电离箱内部离子再结合出现问题时，进行2次电子监控，保证束流强度。再者，要进行定期的基准剂量比的测定，推荐将射野剂量仪的灵敏度变化和监控的敏感度变化同时进行检查。

The dose monitoring system is calibrated by a separate system of two monitors that monitor the dose and monitor the flatness of the field of exposure. Independent beam cutoff signals output from two dose monitors and need to be directly and strictly connected to the respective beam switch. The therapy beam output by pulse. When there is an accident of recombination of ion in the ionizing room, second electric moniting should be taken to ensure the beam intensity. Furthermore, measure the basic dose rate regularly. Recommend check the sensitivity change of the field dosimeter and the monitoring at the same time.

7 患者位置确定 (Patient position determination)

7.1 坐标系精确匹配（Coordinate system exactly matched）

患者位置的确定，是指使用正交的X射线装置（DR），在照射装置上，将患者的PTV设定在等中心位置。等中心位置由两部分决定：从加速器输出的照射系统的束流位置（在照射系统上）以及由准直器确定的照射野中心位置。为了让照射系统上的等中心位置和患者治疗计划上的等中心位置一致，需要对每一位患者做好与照射系统坐标系的精确匹配。

The determination of patient’s position is using irradiation device’s orthogonal X-ray device（DR）to setting the PTV of the patient at the isocenter position. The isocenter position is determined by two parts: The beam position（on the irradiation system）of the irradiation system output from the accelerator and the center position of the field determined by the collimator. In order to align the isocenter position of the irradiation system with the isocenter position of the patient’s therapy plan, each patient needs to be precisely matched to the coordinate system of the irradiation system.

患者位置确定通常遵循以下操作流程。

（1）空间基准坐标系要和束流方向保持一致。

（2）空间基准坐标系要和决定患者位置的X射线装置（DR）的坐标系保持一致。

（3）将患者坐标系和为患者定位的坐标系精确匹配。

评价（1）和（2）阶段的照射系统误差，以及（3）的位置确定操作误差，需要设置边界。以下对照射装置的空间基准坐标系的精度进行说明。首先从治疗室的空间性的坐标系、加速器输出的束流的中心轴来决定。通常，因为束流是以圆锥形发散的，所以准直器位置的误差就会在等中心平面上扩大。因此，位置误差的大小应该在等中心平面上来评价。X射线位置确定装置也同样在等中心进行位置误差的评价。

Patient position determination usually follows the following operation procedure.

(1) The spatial reference coordinate system should be consistent with beam direction.

(2) The spatial reference coordinate system should be consistent with the coordinate system of the X-ray device (DR) that determines the position of the patient.

(3) Precisely match the patient coordinate system with the coordinate system for patient position.

To evaluate the error of irradiation system in stages (1) and (2), and (3)'s operating error in position determination, it is necessary to set the boundary. The accuracy of the spatial reference coordinate system of the irradiation device will be described below. First, it is determined from the spatial coordinate system of the treatment room and the central axis of the beam output from the accelerator. Normally, because the beam is conically divergent, the collimator's position error will expands on the isocenter plane. Therefore, the size of the position error should be evaluated on the isocenter plane. Similarly, the position error of the X - ray position determination device is evaluated at the isocenter.

在使用两个方向X射线图像的患者位置确认操作中，计划系统生成图像（Digitally Reconstructed Radiography，DRR）和在实际照射位置拍摄的X射线图像核对，纠正误差量，调整治疗位置。参照图像和位置确定拍摄图像的特征点坐标的比较等参照相关手册进行操作，或通过图像间的自动比较之类的方法进行。到此，对于显示的目标计算值，如果是在可允许的误差范围之内则可结束操作。

In a patient position confirmation operation using two directional X - ray images, plan system-generated image (Digitally Reconstructed Radiography, DRR) is collated with the X-ray image taken at the actual irradiation position, the error amount thereof is corrected, and the treatment position is adjusted. The comparison of the coordinates of the feature points of the captured image with reference to the image and the position of the captured image may be performed by referring to the related manual or by a method such as automatic comparison between images. At this point, for the displayed target value, the operation can be ended if it is within the allowable error range.

患者固定方面，仰卧位垂直照射或水平照射等照射条件不同时，体位固定方式也有差异。使用摇篮床旋转照射的情况下，固定方法也有很大差异。如果固定具、摇篮床的边缘被包含在照射野里的话，特别是重离子束射程末端位置，它们和患者体位的位置误差会影响剂量分布。因此，制作固定具时，要注意不要将其包含在照射野中。

As for patient fixation, if supine vertical or horizontal irradiation and other irradiation conditions are different, there are differences in immobilization. When using cradle bed rotation irradiation, the immobilization is also very different. If the fixtures, the edge of the cradle bed which are contained in the field of exposure especially at the end of the heavy ion beam range, and the position error of the patient's position affect the dose distribution. Therefore, when making fixtures, do not include them in the field of exposure.

7.2 图像的精确匹配（Exact matching of images）

患者定位时产生的误差，除了照射装置、X射线模拟机坐标产生的误差外，还存在于制作计划时CT图像生产DRR图像时产生的误差。

Besides the errors caused by the irradiation device and X - ray simulator coordinates, the errors that occur when positioning the patient exist in the production of DRR images of the CT images during planning.

数字影像重建图像（DRR）：治疗计划CT生成的DRR图像参数设置要与X射线模拟机的焦点、等中心、投影面等几何学参数一致。这种情况下，DRR的分辨率由三维CT数据的Pixel Spacing（像素间距）、Slice Thickness（层厚）以及DRR生成时*CT*值的内插法、沿着投影轴的计算间隔等决定。有时根据需要也会对*CT*值进行加权处理。

Digitally Reconstructed Radiography（DRR）: The DRR image parameters generated by the treatment plan CT should be the same as those of the X - ray simulator such as the focus, isocenter and projection plane. In this case, the resolution of the DRR is determined by Pixel Spacing, Slice Thickness, and the *CT* value at the time of DRR generation of the three - dimensional CT data, and the calculation interval along the projection axis. *CT* values can sometimes be weighted as needed.

为了确定患者位置，我们需要拍摄一组正交X射线片。成像系统的图像如果是由Image Intensifier（I.I影像增强器）拍摄的话，越接近边缘越会出现扭曲。再者，成像系统的图像也很容易受到地磁影响。近几年，已经普及了可以抑制扭曲的平板探测器。

In order to determine the position of the patient, we need to take a set of orthogonal X - ray radiographs. If the image of the imaging system is taken by Image Intensifier（I.I Image Enhancer), the closer the edge, the more distorted it will appear. In addition, it is also susceptible to geomagnetic effects. In recent years Flat Panel Detecter that can suppress distortion have become popular.

图像比较：DRR图像和X射线正交片比较上，由于影像增强器的拍摄失真、由CT图像生成DRR图像产生失真、拍摄原理的差异，患者固定状态的差异，体型、脏器形状的变化等等，无法取得两张完全一致的图像。在第二次及以后的图像比较上，把第一次拍摄的X射线正交片位置验证图像作为参考图像，用差值运算等方法是可以做到正确的图像比较的。

Image comparison: As for DRR images and X - ray orthogonality, because of the image intensifier shooting distortion, DR images generated by the CT image distortion, differences in shooting principles, the patient's fixed state differences, body shape, organ shape changes etc., we can not get two exactly same image. In the second and later image comparison, the first shot of the X - ray orthogonal position verification image being a reference image, using the difference method, the correct image comparison can be done.

7.3 治疗床（Treatment beds）

治疗床是在患者位置确认时，把患者的靶区中心移动到等中心位置时使用的。包括在位置确定以后不再移动治疗床进行照射和位置确定后、在保证治疗床精度的情况下，移动治疗床进行照射两种情况。

The treatment bed is used when the patient's position is confirmed and the center of the target area of the patient is moved to the isocenter position. The radiotherapy is done by no longer moving the treatment beds when the patient position is fixed and by moving the treatment beds when the accuracy of the treatment bed is ensured if the patient position is fixed.

8 治疗计划系统 (TPS)

在治疗计划系统中，在CT图像上勾画靶区体积以及重要脏器，尽量让高剂量均匀地集中在靶区上，同时重要脏器不要超过允许范围的受量去设定照射野。然后进行重离子治疗装置的设计、补偿器的输出以及体内的剂量分布的计算。

In TPS, the volume of the target area and the important organs are outlined on the CT images, and the high doses are uniformly concentrated on the target area as far as possible while the important organs do not exceed the allowable range to set the irradiation field. The design of the heavy ion therapy device, the output of the compensator, and the calculation of the dose distribution in the body are then performed.

9 *CT*值的水等效厚度转化 (Equivalent water thickness conversion of *CT* value)

离子束在人体内的射程、剂量分布的计算中，需要将*CT*值转化到水等效厚度。这通常是通过对各种各样的组织等效材料的*CT*值以及水等效厚度的测定、计算而求得的。为了保证*CT*值与水等效厚度转化精度，*CT*值的校对、维护是必不可少的。

使用水、肺、肝脏、脂肪、骨等组织等效样本，来测试*CT*值的水等效厚度转化。直接测定样本的*CT*值和水等效厚度，将得出的值进行比较。

CT装置引进时，X射线管、探测器更换等时候，必须使用*CT*值校对模型，把已知测定值和CT图像计算值进行校对。

In calculating the ion beam range in body and dose distribution, the *CT* value needs to be converted to equivalent water thickness. This is usually obtained by measuring and calculating the *CT* values of various tissue equivalent materials and the water equivalent thickness. In order to ensure the *CT* and water equivalent thickness conversion accuracy, *CT* value proofing, maintenance is essential.

Use water, lung, liver, fat, bone and other tissue equivalent samples to test *CT* water equivalent thickness conversion. Measure *CT* value of the sample directly and the water equivalent thickness, and compare them.

When the CT device is introduced, the X-ray tube, the detector is replaced and soon, the *CT* value calibration model must be used to calibrate the known measured value and the calculated value of the CT image.

10 剂量分布计算

(Dose distribution calculation)

剂量计算算法包括射线跟踪法、笔形束法等。采用的算法不同，对离子束散射的计算也不同。较轻的离子束会带来更多的差异。在变更算法、导入新照射法的时候，必须进行剂量分布测量值和计划值的比较。在测定时，剂量仪的体积效果、设置方法、插入剂量仪的模体形状、材质等有很多限制。简单形状的物理模型中的剂量分布可与更为精确的蒙特·卡罗法相比较来评价其精度。

In dose calculation algorithms, there are Ray Tracing, Pencil Beam and so on. Depending on the algorithm, the calculation of the ion beam scattering is also different. The lighter ion beam will bring more difference. When changing the algorithm or introducing a new irradiation method, the dose distribution measurement must be compared with the planned value. In the measurement, there are many restrictions such as the volumetric effect of the dosimeter, setting method, dosimeter body shape inserted, material, etc. The dose distribution in the simple shape of the physical model can be compared with a more accurate Monte Carlo method to evaluate its accuracy.

11 补偿器的制作

(Compensator's production)

补偿器是基于治疗计划系统输出数据，根据数据控制机械来制作的。补偿器的制作精度直接影响束流终端的剂量分布。补偿器的加工精度一般非常好，剂量分布的精度主要由剂量计算的精度决定。但是在深度急剧变化的情况下，可能加工精度不够。可使用其他方法直接测量补偿器加工精度、比较测量值和计划值。要求测量值和计划值的差值不超过±0.5 mm。建议定期检查补偿器材质密度有无变化（测定单位长度的水等效厚度）。

Compensator's production is based on the treatment plan system output data, according to the data control machinery. Compensator production accuracy directly affects the beam end dose distribution. Compensator processing accuracy is generally very good. The accuracy of dose distribution is mainly determined by the accuracy of dose calculation. However, in the case of drastic changes in depth, processing accuracy may not be sufficient. Other methods can be used to measure the compensator machining accuracy directly and to compare measured and planned values. The difference between the measured value and the planned value is required to be less than ± 0.5 mm. It is recommended to regularly check the compensator material density to find whether it changed.（Measure unit length of water equivalent thickness.）

12 呼吸性移动对策

（Countermeasures of respiratory movements）

躯干，特别是肺、肝脏肿瘤的治疗，实行呼吸性移动对策以消除脏器呼吸性移动对照射带来的影响。在JASTRO的呼吸性移动对策指导里记载了很多种方法。呼吸门控中的患者呼吸信号使用压电元件、位置检验型的光电探测器等获得，在某个呼吸位相限制下进行照射。这种情况下，即使是在治疗计划取得CT影像时，也要和实际照射进行同样的呼吸门控。在照射时机方面，对呼吸波形信号设定临界值，规定只在呼吸波形信号临界值以下才可进行照射。也有在特定位相下，经过门信号的密度变化照射的情况。作为重离子治疗中一个特殊的问题，需要在治疗计划设计时考虑束流射程方向靶区的几何学移位以及束流途经中的密度变化。

Torso, especially the lungs, liver tumor treatment need to implement respiratory movement countermeasures to eliminate the impact of respiratory movement of organs. A variety of methods are documented in JASTRO' s Respiratory Movement Countermeasure Guideline. The patient' s breathing signal is got by using a piezoelectric element, a position - based photodetector, etc. The irradiation is done under certain breath - light limitation. In this case, the same gating should be performed as the actual irradiation even when the CT images of the treatment plan are acquired. In terms of timing of exposure, a threshold is set for the respiratory waveform signal to provide exposure only below the threshold of the respiratory waveform signal. There are also cases in which the density of the gate signal changes in a specific phase. As a special issue in heavy ion therapy, it is necessary to consider the geometrical displacement of the target area in the direction of the beam jet and the density change in the beam passage in the design of the treatment plan.

呼吸门控照射误差由以下因素产生：

（1）取得的呼吸波形和实际的脏器移动时的误差。

（2）治疗计划CT图像制作参考图像时的位相不准确。

（3）门控照射下的呼吸波形临界值的设定。

（4）设定门控照射后的有限照射时间下的脏器移动。

Gating error is caused by the following factors:

(1) Errors between respiration waveforms and the actual organ moving.

(2) The phase of the treatment plan CT image when making the reference image is inaccurate.

(3) Gated respiratory wave threshold setting.

(4) Set the organ to move under the limited irradiation time after gating.

13 束流照射范围的误差评价
(Beam irradiation range error evaluation)

需要通过接收测试、日常的质量保证等，掌握设施内束流照射范围的误差，来应对治疗，而且误差应该反映治疗计划设计时设置边界的量。一般情况下，由于照射范围的误差在束流轴方向和束流轴垂直面内不同，所以希望设置边界也根据不同方向使用不同的值。

以下展示束流轴方向和束流轴垂直面内的偶然误差的传播计算示例：

Treatment needs to pass the receiving test, daily QA, etc.. Grasp the scope of the facility within the beam irradiation error. And the error should reflect the amount of boundary that the treatment plan was designed to set. In general, it is desirable to set the boundary and use different values depending on the respective directions because of the difference in irradiation range between the beam axis direction and the beam axis vertical plane.

The following shows an example of calculation of propagation of incidental errors in the direction of the beam axis and in the vertical plane of the beam axis:

13.1 束流行进方向的误差（Error in beam direction）

ΔR：水中的射程误差；

ΔCT：由CT值向水等效厚度转化产生的误差；

ΔF_1：补偿器挖掘精度中纵深方向的误差；

ΔF_2：补偿器材质的误差。

此时，纵深方向的误差（Δd）用以下公式计算：

$$\Delta d = \sqrt{(\Delta R)^2 + (\Delta CT)^2 + (\Delta F_1)^2 + (\Delta F_2)^2}$$

这里导致误差的主要原因是ΔCT。因此，推荐把计算出这个值时的CT值转化水等效厚度的误差限定在2%。

ΔR: Range error in water;

ΔCT: Error resulting from conversion of CT value to water equivalent thickness;

ΔF_1: Error in the depth direction of compensator excavation accuracy;

ΔF_2: Compensator material error.

In this case, the error (Δd) in the depth direction is calculated by the following formular:

$$\Delta d=\sqrt{(\Delta R)^2+(\Delta CT)^2+(\Delta F_1)^2+(\Delta F_2)^2}$$

The main reason for this error is ΔCT. Therefore, it is recommended that when calculating this value, the error of CT equivalent water equivalent thickness is limited to 2%.

13.2 束流轴垂直面内的误差（Errors in the vertical plane of the beam axis）

ΔB：束流轴误差；

ΔC_1：补偿器位置误差；

ΔC_2：对于全照射角度等中心的误差；

ΔX_1：X射线束流轴误差；

ΔX_2：X射线成像系统轴的误差；

ΔP：位置决定演算法的精度；

ΔF_3：患者准直器切削精度。

此时，如果假设各误差间相互独立，垂直面内的误差期待值（ΔW）按下式计算：

$$\Delta W=\sqrt{(\Delta B)^2+(\Delta C_1)^2+(\Delta C)^2+(\Delta X_1)^2+(\Delta X_2)^2+(\Delta P)^2+(\Delta F_3)^2}$$

ΔB: Beam axis error;

ΔC_1: Compensator position error;

ΔC_2: Isocenter error for full angle of illumination;

ΔX_1: X-ray beam axis error;

ΔX_2: Axis error of X-ray imaging system;

ΔP: Location determination algorithm accuracy;

ΔF_3: Patient collimator cutting accuracy;

In this case, the expected error value (ΔW) in the vertical plane is calculated as follows, assuming that the errors are independent of each other:

$$\Delta W=\sqrt{(\Delta B)^2+(\Delta C_1)^2+(\Delta C)^2+(\Delta X_1)^2+(\Delta X_2)^2+(\Delta P)^2+(\Delta F_3)^2}$$

14 重离子治疗装置的维护保养（Heavy ion therapy device maintenance）

为了保证离子束治疗装置的精度，需要进行定期的维护保养。以下叙述装置厂家参与的应该进行的维护保养内容。如果由于离子束流治疗装置的技术有其他革新，或自动控制等方法能进行确保的话，以下内容可以不使用。

To ensure the accuracy of the ion beam treatment device, regular maintenance is required. The following is the necessary maintenance the equipment manufacturers should participate. If there is any other innovation due to the technology of the ion beam therapy device, or automatic control, etc., the following can not be used.

15 治疗束流检查

（Beam inspection）

治疗束流非常重要的是，完全按照治疗计划中的核素、能量，特别是拥有多个治疗室的情况下，需要保持束流特性的重复性。因此，日常的QA中，确保束流特性的同时，根据机头内的束流监控在照射中也要随时监视，超出规定值时需要立刻停止束流。此外，还有在实施治疗之前进行确认、照射少量束流来确认束流特性等方法。

It is very important that beam flow should be completely in accordance with the treatment plan of nuclides, energy, especially with multiple treatment rooms to maintain the repeatability of beam characteristics. Therefore, in the daily QA, the beam characteristics should be ensured as well as the beam current monitoring in the handpiece should be monitored at any time. When beam exceed the specified value, the beam should be stopped immediately. In addition, there are methods of confirming the beam current before confirming the treatment and confirming the beam current characteristics.

16 剂量监控系统的检查

（Dose monitoring system inspection）

进行基准条件下深部剂量分布测量以及固定点的剂量测量，检查*MU*值剂量变化、射程变化。确认据此加速的离子是规定的核素、规定的能量。剂量监控以及其他装置也要确认离子束流治疗装置正常运转。

Measure the deep dose distribution and the fixed point dose, check *MU* dose changes, range changes under the reference conditions. Confirm that the accelerated ion according to this is a predetermined nuclide, the prescribed energy. As for dose monitoring and other devices, the ion beam therapy device also should be confirmed to be functioning properly.

17 照射野平坦度的检查

（Radiation field flatness inspection）

取基准照射条件下的SOBP中心处的横切面剂量分布，确认此时的平坦度是规定的精度。这些有关重复性的确认需要建立自己的方案。重离子治疗装置需要有日常检查照射野的平坦度的功能以确保实现照射野平坦度监控的重复性和稳定性。

Select the cross - sectional dose distribution at the SOBP center under baseline exposure conditions. Confirm that the flatness at this time is the prescribed accuracy. Programs about these repetitive confirmations need to established. Heavy ion therapy devices require the ability of routinely checking the flatness of the radiation field to ensure repeatability and stability of radiation field flatness monitoring.

18 束流以及位置决定调整

(Beam and position decision adjustments)

固定口的情况：

进行扩大束流照射时，束流轴最终是由束流扩大焦点和补偿器的位置来决定的。观察、调整束流轴和患者在X射线影像系统中的位置就可以在规定位置安装补偿器托架，再根据束流照射和依据X射线照射二次曝光，即可测量各自的照射野中心在X射线胶片上的偏差。束流中心轴可以根据固定在重离子治疗装置上的“十”字金属丝的X射线图像上的位置来判断。

位置决定大多都在FPD上及I.I.上进行。必须把成像仪的中心设定在X射线轴的中心，设置成几何学束流线的十字线用X射线曝光，其影子作为中心。

Fixed export situation:

When expanding beam irradiation, the beam axis is ultimately determined by the beam expanding focal point and compensator position. After observing and adjusting the position of the beam axis and the patient in the X-ray imaging system, the compensator bracket can be installed at a specified position. Then according to beam irradiation and secondary exposure of X-ray irradiation, you can measure the deviation of the center of each irradiation field in X-ray film. The beam center axis can be determined by the X-ray image position of the shape metal wire attached to the heavy ion therapy device.

The position decision is mostly on the FPD and I.I. The center of the imager must be set at the center of the X-ray axis and the crosshairs, which are set to geometrically beam lines, are exposed by the X-ray with the shadow being the center.

19 呼吸门控装置的动作

(Movement of gating device)

呼吸门控的时机，需要与治疗计划使用的图像一致。将门控级别的调整尽量重现出来，切实按照呼吸门控照射的进行。

The timing of respiration gating needs to be consistent with the images used in the treatment plan. The gating level adjustments should be as far as possible to reproduce, in strict accordance with respiratory gating control.

20 剂量计算

(Dose calculation)

剂量计算精度的确认一定要在接收测试、治疗计划变更时进行。定期进行检查也非常重要。确认工作可以分成两类：一个是，确认剂量计算的基准、确认瞄准照射体积的计算以及确认与登记的数据比较；另一个是，确认不均匀性介质中或补偿器方面的计算。

Confirmation of the dose calculation accuracy must be done when receive test, change treatment plan. Regular inspection is also very important. Confirmation work can be divided into two categories: one is to confirm the basis of the dose calculation, the calculation for the targeting irradiation volume, and the confirmation, compared to the registered data. The other is to confirm the calculation in the non-uniform medium or in the compensator.

20.1 标准照射体积的确认（无补偿器）

［Confirmation of standard irradiation volume （without compensator）］

使用水模体，多叶准直器按照以下条件的组合进行：

（1）标准照射体积下照射野尺寸和SOBP宽度，取被使用范围内的标准条件、极端大的条件、极端小的条件三种条件。

（2）束流能量使用全部能量，射程移位器的值按照各能量分别取大、中、小三种。

Using a water phantom, a multi-leaf collimator is used in combination with the following conditions:

（1）The irradiation field size and the SOBP width under the standard irradiation volume are taken as the standard conditions, the extremely large conditions and the extremely small conditions within the used range.

（2）Beam energy use all the energy, and the value of the range shifter in accordance with the energy are taken large, medium and small.

20.2 模拟治疗束流（有补偿器）［Simulated treatment beam （with compensator）］

（1）在水模体中放入具有与水不同*CT*值的物质（肺等效以及骨等效），设定适当的靶区，设计治疗计划。

（2）基于治疗计划制作补偿器。

（3）靶区设定为几何学的形状。

（1）Place substances with *CT* values different from water in the water phantom（lung equivalent and bone equivalent）, set appropriate targets and design treatment plans.

（2）Make compensator based on treatment plan.

（3）The target area is set to a geometric shape.

21 装置的QA项目和容许值

（QA project and tolerance of device）

除了厂家参与的保养管理以外，下面叙述装置使用者应该进行的QA项目。本指导方针推荐实施的装置QA项目分为以下五个范畴：

（1）剂量仪：有关治疗束流输出管理的项目。

（2）几何学部分：有关装置、患者的位置匹配、照射野的形成的项目。

（3）位置核查系统：有关患者位置匹配时使用的图像装置的项目。

（4）呼吸门控系统：进行呼吸门控时必需的项目。

（5）安全装置系统：连锁等安全装置的项目。

In addition to the manufacturer's maintenance management, the following describes the QA items that device users should conduct. The QA project recommended by this guideline is divided into the following five categories:

(1) Dosimeter: Items of managing the output of beam.

(2) Geometry Department: Items of device, the patient's position matching, the formation of irradiation field.

(3) Location verification system: Items related to the image device used when the patient position is matched.

(4) Gating control system: respiratory gating necessary items.

(5) Safety devices: Items of interlocks and other safety devices.

上述项目各自以不同频率在有关QA项目中显示其说明和容许值。容许值显示了调查级别和即时应对级别两个值。但是，因为有指导方针，所以只记录一般项目。实际具体的测量方法、频率、容许值、应对方法，最终都应该由机构来决定。机构内医生、物理师为核心的医疗工作人员，在充分理解重离子治疗装置所要求的性能、治疗精度基础之上，根据需要设计并运用适合本机构的QA项目。

Each of these items shows its description and tolerances in the relevant QA project on a different frequency. The allowable value shows both the investigation level and the immediate response level. However, because of the guidelines, only the general items were recorded. The actual specific measurement method, frequency, allowable value and coping method should all be decided by the agency. The doctors and physicians are the core medical staff. When fully understanding the demanded quality and accuracy of the heavy ion therapy device, design and apply QA project for the agency according to the need.

QA项目筹划的时候，和各自的保养管理项目核对，追加相应QA项目，提高频率，将容许值严格化。在经过充分讨论的情况下，可以把被判断为低优先度的项目降低频率。

有关容许值和测量值的测量精度，要调查是否在一个容许值内，一般要求在这个容许值一半以下范围内。有关重离子束流的QA，只把物理吸收剂量作为对象。这里显示的容许值意思是“±N%”的数值。例如，在容许值是1%时和基线的差进行比较，把测量值设为m，基线值设为B，其误差量d用以下方法计算：

$$d=\left(1-\frac{m}{B}\right)\times 100\%$$

这里的d值在±1%以内则判定为合格。如果重复测量了，就用测量值的平均值来判定。

When QA projects are planned, QA items should be added with the respective maintenance management items, increase the frequency, and allow the values to be more stringent. After sufficient discussion, the frequency of projects judged as low priority can be reduced.

The tolerances and measurement accuracy, are generally required to be within half the allowable value, check them to see if they are within an allowable value. QA for heavy ion beam only targets physically absorbed doses. The tolerance shown here means "±N%". For example, when the allowable value is 1%, the difference from the baseline is compared, the measured value is set to be m, the baseline value is set to be B, and the error amount d is calculated as follows:

$$d=\left(1-\frac{m}{B}\right)\times 100\%$$

Here, if the value of d is within ±1%, it can be judged as acceptable. If you repeat the measurements, use the average of the measurements to make the decision.

22 剂量仪
(Dosimeter)

频率	项目	即时应对级别容许值	调查级别容许值
每天	输出的稳定性(Output stability)	2%	1%
〃	副剂量监控的稳定性(Side dose monitoring stability)	2%	1%
每月	输出的稳定性(Output stability)	2%	1%
〃	轴外剂量比的稳定性(Off-axis dose ratio stability)	1%	0.5%
〃	射程的稳定性(Range stability)	1 mm	0.5 mm
每年	平坦度的变化(Flatness changes)	1%	0.5%
〃	对称性的变化(Symmetry changes)	2%	1%
〃	监控剂量仪的校对(Monitor dosimeter calibration)	1%	0.5%
〃	监控的直线性(Linearity of Monitoring)	2%	0.5%
〃	输出稳定性的剂量率依赖性(Dose rate dependent of output stability)	2%	0.5%
〃	百分深度剂量(PDD)的测量和基准的差[(PDD) measurement and the reference difference]	2%	1%
〃	SOBP内的平坦度(绝对值)[SOBP flatness (absolute value)]		3%

22.1　每天的项目（Daily Items）

·输出的稳定性（Output stability）

正常测量条件下，测量射野剂量仪输出和剂量监控/计数的比（Gy/count），检查与上次的监控剂量仪比较时的测量结果的差是否在容许值以内。

Under normal measurement conditions, measure the ratio of output of the dosimeter to dose monitor / count (Gy / count) to see if the difference in measurement results from the previous monitor dosimeter is within allowable value.

·副剂量监控的稳定性（side dose monitoring stability）

正常测量条件下，测量射野剂量仪输出和副剂量监控/计数的比（Gy/count），检查与上次的监控剂量仪比较时的测量结果的差是否在容许值以内。

Under normal measurement conditions, measure the ratio of the output of the dosimeter to side dose monitor / count (Gy / count) to see if the difference in measurement results from the previous monitor dosimeter is within allowable value.

22.2　每月的项目（Monthly Items）

·输出的稳定性（Output stability）

在治疗时使用频率高的代表性能量测量条件下，测量射野剂量仪输出和剂量监控/计数的比（Gy/count），检查与上次测量结果的差是否在容许值以内。关于比日常测量条件多的束流测量条件，希望能用更高精度来测量。

Under the measurement condition of the representative energy with high frequency during treatment, measure the ratio of output of the dosimeter to dose monitoring / counting (Gy / count) to see if the difference from the last measurement is within the allowable value. More beam measurement conditions than usual are expected to be measured with higher accuracy.

·轴外剂量比的稳定性（Off-axis dose ratio stability）

在正常测量条件下，基准深度测量4个以上点的束流轴和垂直平面上照射野内的轴外剂量比（OCR），检查各测量点差的平均值是否在容许值内。轴外剂量比的定义是，某个位置的剂量与同一深度的束流轴上的剂量的比值。

Under normal measurement conditions, the baseline depth measures the off-axis dose-to-volume ratio (OCR) over the beam axis of more than 4 points and the vertical field, and check whether the average of each measurement point difference is within the allowable value. The off-axis dose ratio is defined as the ratio of the dose at one location to the dose at the beam axis at the same depth.

· 射程的稳定性（Range stability）

对于治疗中使用的全部能量，测量笔形束流或者代表性的束流条件的射程，检查其与基线的差是否在容许值内。希望能用可以调节电离室深度的水模体来测量深度剂量分布。纵深方向照射成像板或用几个深度下的剂量测量来推断射程等方法也是很好的。

For all the energy used in the treatment, measure the range of pen beam or representative beam conditions and check if the difference from baseline is within allowable value. It is desirable to measure the depth dose distribution with a water phantom that can adjust the depth of the ionization chamber. It is also good practice to illuminate the imaging plate in the depth direction or to dose range with several depth measurements to infer the range.

22.3　每年的项目（Annual Items）

· 平坦度的变化（Flatness changes）

正常测量条件下，测量对*X*轴和*Y*轴的OCR，检查它们的平坦度和基线的差是否在容许值内。最好使用二维扫描测量的电离室。通过二维探测器、成像板测量也很好。

Under normal measurement conditions, measure the OCRs on the *X* - axis and the *Y* - axis to see if their flatness and baseline difference are within allowable values. It is best to use ionization chambers for 2D scanning measurements. Through the two - dimensional detector, imaging plate measurement is also very good.

· 对称性的变化（Symmetry changes）

在日常测量条件下，测量对*X*轴和*Y*轴的OCR，确认它们的对称性和基线的差是否在容许值内。最好使用二维扫描测量的电离箱。通过二维探测器、成像板测量也好。

Under normal measurement conditions, measure the OCRs on the *X* - axis and the *Y* - axis and verify that their symmetry and baseline difference are within acceptable values. It is best to use a two - dimensional scanning ionization chamber. Through the two - dimensional detector, imaging plate measurement is also very good.

· 监控剂量仪的校对（Monitor dosimeter calibration）

正常测量条件下，遵循标准测量法，测量水吸收剂量绝对值，检查和基线的差是否在容许值内。如超出容许值的情况下，检查监控剂量仪的校对常数。

Under normal measurement conditions, follow the standard measurement method to measure the absolute value of water absorbed dose to confirm whether the difference from the baseline is within the allowable value. If the permissible value is exceeded, check the calibration constant of the dosimeter.

· 监控的直线性（Linearity of monitor）

正常测量条件下，测量射野剂量仪输出和剂量监控/计数比（Gy/count）对剂量监控/计数的依赖性，检查它的变化在一次治疗照射剂量范围下是否在容许值内。

Under normal measurement conditions, measure the dependence of dosimeter output and dose monitoring / count ratio（D / C）on dose monitoring / counting to check whether its change is within allowable value for a single dose of therapeutic radiation.

· 输出稳定性的剂量率依赖性（Dose rate dependent of output stability）

正常测量条件下，剂量率和治疗时不同时（如果在可以调整的范围内则不进行），测量射野剂量仪输出和与剂量监控/计数的比（Gy/count），检查与治疗时的剂量率测量值的差是否在容许值范围内。

Under normal measurement conditions, if the dose rate is different from that at the time of treatment（measurement if it is within the adjustable range）, measure the output of the dosimeter and the ratio（Gy / count）to the dose monitoring / count, check whether the difference between the dose rate measurements is within the allowable range.

· 百分深度剂量（PDD）的测量和基准的差［（PDD）measurement and the reference difference］

治疗使用的代表性束流条件下，测量百分深度剂量（PDD），检查和基线的差是否在容许值内。射程附近重离子线的情况下，间隔0.5 mm以内进行测量。希望射程移位器（Range Shifter）的水等效厚度能够一并确认。

Under typical beam conditions for therapeutic use, measure the percentage depth dose（PDD）, check whether is measured to confirm the difference from the baseline is within tolerance. In the case of heavy ion lines near the range, the measurement is performed within 0.5 mm intervals. It is hoped that the water equivalent thickness, including the Range Shifter, will be confirmed together.

· SOBP内平坦度（绝对值）［SOBP flatness （absolute value）］

治疗使用的代表性束流条件下，测量SOBP内的OCR，确认平坦度的绝对值在容许值内。

Under typical beam conditions for treatment, measure the OCR in the SOBP, confirm that the absolute value of the flatness was within the allowable value.

23 几何学系

(Geometry)

几何学系的QA项目（Geometric QA project）

频率	项目		即时应对级别容许值	调查级别容许值
每天	激光位置(Laser position)		1.5 mm	1 mm
〃	多叶准直器开口时叶片位置(MLC leaf position when opening)		1 mm	0.5 mm
每月	十字线中心位置(Cross center position)		2%	1%
〃	治疗床位置(Position of the couch)	平行移动 旋转角度	1 mm 1°	0.5 mm 0.5°
〃	补偿器位置(Compensator position)		1 mm	0.5 mm
〃	准直器角度(Collimator angle)		1°	0.5°
每年	束流等中心位置(Beam isocenter position)		2 mm	1 mm
〃	束流中心和X射线图像中心的一致(Beam center and X-ray image center consistency)		2 mm	1.5 mm
〃	治疗床的等中心位置(由半径判定)(Bed isocenter position)		2%	1.5 mm
〃	治疗床的弯曲度(Curvature of the bed)		2 mm	1%
〃	治疗床最大移动距离(Maximum movement of the treatment bed)		2 mm	1 mm
〃	SOBP过滤器外观(SOBP filter appearance)		没有异常	
〃	射程移位器外观(Range shifter appearance)		没有异常	
〃	Snout位置(Snout location)		2 mm	1 mm
〃	十字线中心位置(基准点)[Cross center position (reference point)]		1 mm	0.5 mm

23.1 每天的项目（Daily items）

· 激光位置（Laser position）

根据在机器上的标记，或者被设置在标准位置的目标物体，检查等中心的激光位置误差是否在容许值内。如果在表示同一轴的多个激光的情况下，也要检查它们之间有无差别。

Check whether the laser position error of the isocenter is within the allowable value based on the mark on the machine or the target object set at the standard position. If you are in the same axis of multiple laser case, check whether there is any difference between them also.

· 多叶准直器开口时叶片位置（MLC leaf position when opening）

在多叶准直器适当开口时测量叶片位置，检查与设定值的差是否在容许值内。如果直接测量困难的话，用光照射野、X射线图像等间接确认也可以。

When MLC is properly open, measure the leaf position and check whether the difference from the set value is within the allowable value. If it is difficult to measure between them directly, confirm by light exposure field, X-ray image, etc. indirectly is acceptable.

23.2 每月的项目（Monthly Items）

· 十字线中心位置（Cross center position）

检查激光中心和十字线中心的误差是否在容许值内。

旋转准直器，检查十字线中心是否偏离中心。同时，至少一年一次，基于建筑物上或者固定在建筑物上的装置上的基准点确认十字线中心位置。

Check the laser center and cross center error whether they are within tolerance.

Turn the collimator to check that whether the center of the crosshair is off center. Also, at least once a year, confirm the centerline of the crosshair based on a reference point on the building or on a fixture attached to the building.

· 治疗床位置（Position of the couch）

使用规尺、治疗床的刻度或模型的X射线图像等，检查治疗床的移动量、旋转角度在表示值和容许值内是否一致。

Using the scale, the scale of the couch, the X-ray image of the model, or the like, check whether the amount of movement and the rotation angle of the couch are the same between the indicated value and the allowable value.

· 补偿器位置（Compensator position）

检查补偿器的安装位置是否在容许值内。也可以在中心附近使用刻度、带标记的补偿器代替物等进行光学测量。

Check whether the installation position of the compensator is within the allowable value. It is also acceptable to use optical scales near the center, optically compensated markers, etc.

· 准直器角度（Collimator angle）

使用角度计等测量准直器的旋转角度，确认表示值和误差在容许值内是否一致。

Use an angle meter or the like to measure the angle of rotation of the collimator to check whether the indication value and the error agree is the same within the allowable value.

23.3 每年的项目（Annual items）

· 束流等中心位置（Beam isocenter position）

直接或间接测量束流等中心（相当于重离子束流Radiation isocenter）和建筑上基线位置的关系，检查与基线位置的距离在容许值内是否一致。例如，使用X射线胶片，根据准直器旋转进行Starshot，把交点重心位置作为束流等中心。如果知道激光中心和基线位置的关系，就可以测量X射线胶片上的束流等中心和基线位置的距离。

Directly or indirectly measure the isocenter of the beam （equivalent to heavy ion beam Radiation isocenter） and the relationship between the construction of the baseline position to check the distance from the baseline position within the allowable value is consistent. For example, using X-ray film, the Starshot is rotated according to the collimator, and the center of gravity of the point of intersection is used as the center of the beam. If you know the location of the laser center and the baseline position, you can measure the distance between the beam center and the baseline position on the X-ray film.

· 束流中心和X射线图像中心的一致（Beam center and X-ray image center consistency）

直接或间接检查束流中心（根据准直器制作的照射野中心）和X射线图像中心的距离在容许值内是否一致。例如，在X射线图像中心设置金属球，直接或间接地测量束流产生的剂量分布内的金属球影子中心位置和束流中心的位置关系。如果直接测量很难的话，让激光等介入，测量相对激光中心的束流中心位置和相对激光中心的X射线图像中心位置，再由各自的位置关系算出。

Check directly or indirectly whether the distance between the beam center （based on the center of irradiation field of the collimator） and the X-ray image center is within the allowable value. For example, a metal ball is set at the center of the X-ray image to directly or indirectly measure the position relationship between the center position of the metal ball and the beam center in the dose distribution caused by the beam current. If the direct measurement is difficult, let the laser and other intervention, relative to the center of the laser beam center and relative to the laser center of the X-ray image center position, and then from their positional relationship, the distance can be calculated.

· 治疗床的等中心位置（Bed isocenter position）

位置匹配时，对于等中心靶区位置，检查三维照射计划的治疗床移动后的靶区位置是否在容许值内。从设置在治疗床的目标物的位置和激光等的关系测量相对移动量。

When match the positions, for the isocenter target position, check whether the position of the target moved by the three-dimensional irradiation plan bed is within the allowable value. The amount of relative movement is measured from the relationship between the position of the target placed on the couch bed and laser light.

· 治疗床的弯曲度（Curvature of the bed）

日本工业规格JIS-4714（中国根据国家食品药品监督管理总局发布的《质子/碳离子治疗系统技术审查指导原则》，床面的横向刚度要求参考IEC62667）作为参考，把对应患者的标准负重放在治疗床上，用卷尺、激光距离计等测量弯曲量。检查弯曲量的基线差是否在容许值内。

Japanese Industrial Specifications JIS-4714（according to the *Guidelines for Technical*

Review of Proton/ Carbon Ion Therapy Systems published by the State Food and Drug Administration in China, reference for lateral rigidity of the bed Reference IEC62667）as reference, place the standard weight of the corresponding patient on the couch, measure the amount of bending with a tape measure, a laser distance meter, or the like. Check whether the baseline amount of deflection is within the allowable value.

· 治疗床的最大移动距离（Maximum bed movement distance）

检查治疗床的最大移动位置的再现性是否在容许值内。测量最大移动距离位置和治疗室标记的关系。

Check whether the reproducibility of the maximum movement position of the couch is within the allowable value. Measure the relationship between the location of the maximum distance of movement and the mark of the treatment room.

· SOBP过滤器的外观（SOBP filter appearance）

肉眼检查所有的SOBP过滤器（脊型过滤器）有没有扭曲、伤痕等。检查过滤器ID等是否能正确识别、是否设置在规定位置。

Visual inspection check whether all SOBP filters（ridge filters）have distortion, scratches, etc. Check whether the ID of the filter can be correctly recognized and set in the specified position.

· 射程移位器的外观（Range shifter appearance）

检查是否有扭曲、伤痕。检查是否设置在规定位置。

Check whether there is distortion, scar. Check whether it is set at the specified position.

· Snout的位置（Snout's location）

运用Snout的位置规定、encoder等，检查Snout的移动量以及Snout的移动轴在束流轴上是否在容许值内。

Using Snout's position specification, encoder, etc., check whether the movement amount of Snout and the movement axis of Snout are within the allowable value on the beam axis.

· 十字线中心位置（基准点）[Cross center position （reference point）]

将建筑或被固定在建筑上构造物的标记作为基准，检查和十字线中心的误差是否在容许值内。

Using the mark of the building or the structure to be fixed on the building as a reference, check whether the error from the center of the crosshair is within the allowable value.

24 位置核查

(Location verification)

位置核查的QA项目

频率	项目	即时应对级别容许值	调查级别容许值
每天	X射线图形表示坐标(X-ray image coordinates)	1 mm	0.5 mm
〃	X射线图像中心和激光中心一致(X-ray image center and laser center of consistency)	2 mm	1 mm
每月	刻度的精度(Accuracy of the scale)	2 mm	1 mm
〃	图像扭曲补正(Image distortion correction)	和基线的差很小	
〃	画质确认(Quality confirmation)	和基线的差很小	
〃	X射线种类确认(X-ray type confirmation)	和基线的差很小	
〃	辐射剂量(Radiation dose)	和基线的差很小	

24.1 每天的项目 (Daily items)

· X射线图像表示坐标 (X-ray image coordinates)

检查X射线图像表示画面上的原点和Snout十字线影的中心距离是否在容许值内。检查X射线图像表示画面的坐标轴是否倾斜。

Check whether the distance between the origin on the X-ray image display screen and the center of the Snout cross-hair shadow is within the allowable value. Check whether the X-ray image indicates that the axis of the screen is tilted.

· X射线图像中心和激光中心的一致 (X-ray image center and laser center of consistency)

把金属球的中心、金属线交点设置成和激光中心一致，检查和X射线图像中心的误差是否在容许值内。而且，一年一次，要正确把握建筑物、机架的X射线图像中心的位置精度。

The center of the metal ball and the intersection of the metal line are set to coincide with the laser center, check whether the X-ray image center error is within allowable value. What's more, once a year, it is necessary to correctly grasp the positional accuracy of the X-ray image center of a building or a rack.

24.2　每月的项目（Monthly items）

·刻度的精度（Accuracy of the scale）

在规定的间隔设置金属球或金属线，拍摄X射线图像，检查画面上测量的距离和设置间隔是否在容许值内。

Set metal balls or metal wires at specified intervals and take X-ray images, check whether the distance measured on the screen and the setting interval are within the allowable values.

24.3　每年的项目（Annual items）

·图像扭曲的补正（Image distortion correction）

使用I.I.管的X射线位置确定图像装置的情况下，使用测量扭曲的器具（grit型线等），确认扭曲，确认与基线的差很小。

In the case of using the X-ray position of the I.I. tube to determine the image device, use a measuring instrument （grit type wire, etc.） to confirm the distortion and confirm that the difference from the baseline is small.

·画质确认

确认X射线图像的对比、空间分辨能力、均一性、噪音等与基线的差很小。

Confirm X-ray image contrast, spatial resolution, uniformity, noise and other differences from the baseline are small.

·X射线种类确认（X-ray type confirmation）

测量半价层（Half Value Layer：HVL），确认与基线的偏差很小。

Measure the Half Value Layer （HVL） and confirm that the deviation from the baseline is small.

·辐射剂量（Radiation dose）

使用正交2野的X射线装置时，进行入射表面剂量的测量等，确认和基线的差很小。

When using an orthogonal 2-field X-ray apparatus, measurement of the incident surface dose and the like were performed, and the difference from the baseline was confirmed to be small.

25 呼吸门控

（Respiratory gating）

呼吸门控的QA项目（QA items of respiratory gating）

频率	项目	即时应对级别容许值	调查级别容许值
每月	出束的稳定性（Stability of beam）	2%	1%
〃	呼吸相位、振幅束流控制（Respiratory phase, amplitude beam control）	动作确认	动作确认
〃	室内呼吸监控系统（Indoor respiratory monitoring system）	动作确认	动作确认
〃	门控的连锁（Interlock of gate）	动作确认	动作确认
每年	射程稳定性（Stability of range）	1 mm	0.5 mm
〃	门控开/关、束流开/关的时间精度（Time accuracy of gate on / off and beam on / off）	50 ms	25 ms
〃	相位振幅门控打开时间精度（Time accuracy of phase / amplitude gate on）	100 ms	100 ms
〃	相位振幅的代替物的校正（Correction of phase / amplitude substitutes）	100 ms	100 ms
〃	连锁测试（Interlock test）	动作确认	动作确认

25.1 每月的项目（Monthly Items）

·出束的稳定性（Stability of beam）

在日常测量的同等条件下，测量呼吸门控系统gate on/off状态。这时候，呼吸模拟波形、gate on/off条件，采用和实际质量相近的。与反复测量取得的再现性、无呼吸门控下的照射进行比较，检查输出的稳定性是否在容许值内。在AAPM-TG142报告中推荐使用动态模型，但是为了验证加速器装置，在模拟波形上gate on/off使用静止模型测量剂量也是可以的。

Under the same conditions of daily measurement, measure the gate on / off state of the respiratory gating system. At this time, breathing simulation waveforms, gate on / off conditions, are similar to the actual quality. The repeatability obtained by repeated measurements and the irradiation without breath gating are compared to check whether the stability of the output is within the allowable value. A dynamic model is recommended for use in the AAPM-TG142 report, but in order to verify the accelerator device, it is also possible to use a static model to measure the dose of the gate on / off on the analog waveform.

·呼吸位相、振幅束流控制（Respiratory phase, amplitude beam control）

呼吸门控系统和呼吸波形同步，让gate on/off信号输出，检查束流是否输出。为了确认波形输出后装置的完好性，用模拟波形也可以。

Respiratory gating system and respiratory waveform synchronization, the gate on / off signal output to check whether the beam output. To confirm the integrity of the device after the waveform is output, it is also possible to use an analog waveform.

· 室内呼吸监控系统（Indoor respiratory monitoring system）

在呼吸门控监控画面上检查呼吸门控系统的传感器等是否正常运作。

Check the sensors of respiratory gating system function properly on the respiratory gating monitoring screen .

· 门控的连锁（Interlock of gate）

按下呼吸门控系统装备的手动gate off按钮时，确认gate从on变到了off。

When pressing the manual gate off button equipped with the respiration gating system, confirm that the gate has changed from on to off.

25.2　每年的项目（Annual items）

· 射程稳定性（Stability of range）

检查呼吸门控模式的束流射程和通常模式（非门控）的束流射程是否一致。确认方法遵循通常模式下射程确认方法。

Check whether beam range of the respiratory gated mode matches that of the normal mode (not gated). Confirm that the method follow the normal mode range confirmation method.

· 门控开/关和束流开/关的时间精度（Time accuracy of gate on / off and beam on / off）

把呼吸门控系统模拟波形下的从gate on/off信号到束流产生/停止的延迟时间、gate on信号和束流监控信号输入示波镜并测量，检查束流关是否在容许值内。脊型过滤器的情况下，有关束流开的重要度低，所以不设定容许值也可以。但就三维的照射野形成方法（脊型过滤器、Wabbling周波数、螺旋Wabbling等扫描方法），为了获得均一的照射野，必要的gate和束流on/off的逻辑、精度需要依据设施内机器设定容许值。

The delay time, the gate on signal, the beam monitoring signal from the gate on / off signal, to the beam generation / stop, are input to the scope for measurement under the analog waveform of the respiratory gating system, check whether the beam off is within the allowable value. In the case of the ridge filter, the degree of importance of the beam opening is low, so the allowable value is not set. However, for the three - dimensional radiation field formation method (ridge filter, Wabbling frequency, spiral Wabbling and other scanning methods), in order to obtain a uniform radiation field, the logic and accuracy of the necessary gate and beam on / off allowable value should be set according to the machine in the facility.

［基准值并不是一个绝对的东西，在把握每个设备（site - specific & technique -

specific）的特征情况下，把它们都考虑进去再制订治疗计划、治疗是非常重要的。]

(The base value is not an absolute thing. It is important to take each of them into account and then plan the treatment and treat, when the site-specific & technique-specific features are grasped.)

· 相位/振幅门控打开时间精度（Time accuracy of phase / amplitude gate on）

测量从模拟波形的相位/振幅到gate on信号输出的延迟时间，检查是否在容许值内。

[【100ms】的时间精度，假设时间不超过20 ms，预测结果应该在2 mm的位置精度上。]

Measure the delay time from the phase / amplitude of the analog waveform to the gate on signal output, check whether it is within the allowable value.

(As for [100ms] time accuracy, assuming that the time does not exceed 20 ms, the position accuracy of the prediction results should be 2 mm position accuracy.)

· 相位/振幅的代替物的校正（Correction of phase / amplitude substitutes）

确认代替物的变化（查出位置的动作、压力变化、换气量变化等）和得到的波形关系（变位、时间）的再现。例如从动体模型得到呼吸波形的时候，确认模型动作和波形的振幅、时机的再现。振幅的确认是，测量某个决定动量的模型，检查用同样的设定（扩大率）能否得到同样的呼吸波形。时机的确认方法，可以是拍摄模型动作和波形一起的动画。通过用示波镜测量等方法，确认相当于模型动作的波形和输出的呼吸波形。但是，测量方法是由各机构来决定的，目的是确认接收时的再现性。

Confirm the change of the substitute (operation of the detected position, change of pressure, change of the amount of ventilation, etc.) and reproduction of the obtained waveform relation (displacement, time). For example, when a respiratory waveform is obtained from a moving body model, the model motion and the amplitude and timing of the waveform are confirmed. The confirmation of the amplitude is to measure a certain momentum model and check whether the same respiratory waveform can be obtained with the same setting (magnification). The method of how to recognize the timing, may be taking animations with model actions and waveforms. Confirm the waveform corresponding to the model operation and the output respiratory waveform by using the oscilloscope measurement and other methods. However, the measurement method is determined by each agency in order to confirm the reproducibility of reception.

· 连锁试验（Interlock test）

有关呼吸门控照射中如果发生什么事故时，束流可以立刻切断的相关事宜，要模拟事故进行确认。模拟事故的具体方法有，例如强制停止呼吸门控控制软件或拔掉电缆确认束流停止等方法。希望各机构可以考虑到自己的照射装置、呼吸门控装置的构成来决定。

In the event of respiratory gating irradiation incident, the related issues that the beam can be immediately cut off can be confirmed by simulating the incident to confirm. Specific methods of simulating an accident include, for example, forcing the respiratory gated control software to stop, or unplugging the cable to confirm that the beam is stopped. It is hoped that agencies can take into account the composition of their own irradiation devices and respiratory gating devices.

26 安全装置

(Safety device)

安全装置的QA项目（QA items of Safety device）

频率	项目	容许值
每天	门连锁(Door interlock)	运作确认
〃	门开关途中的安全性(Door switch safety on the way)	运作确认
〃	声音、图像监控(Sound and image monitoring)	运作确认
〃	放射线区域监控(Radiation area monitoring)	运作确认
〃	束流 on 表示(Beam on display)	运作确认
〃	Snout 冲突连锁(Snout conflict interlock)	运作确认
〃	X射线装置冲突连锁(X-ray device conflict interlock)	运作确认
〃	患者用呼叫按钮(Patient call button)	运作确认
每年	紧急停止结构的运作确认(Emergency stop switch operation confirmation)	运作确认

26.1 每天的项目（Daily Items）

· 门连锁（Door interlock）

确认在门开着的状态下是不出束的。

Make sure that the door is open without a beam.

· 门开关途中的安全性（Door switch safety on the way）

确认治疗室门开关途中的安全性。例如如果是关门途中有东西进入、传感器有反应并停止门的动作这种设计的话，确认它。

Confirm the safety of the treatment room door switch on the way. Confirm such design, for example, if there is something on the way to the door and the sensor reacts and stops the door.

· 声音、图像监控（Sound and image monitoring）

声音监控：进行对讲机的运作（音量、音质）确认。评价从操作室到治疗室内声音的听取、从治疗室到操作室内声音的听取。确认监控像机的运作范围、旋转、镜头、焦距调整功能。

Sound Monitor: Confirm the operation of radio (volume, sound quality). Listen to the sound from the operating room to the treatment room and listen to the sound from the treatment room to the operating room. Confirm the monitoring camera's operating range, rotation, lens, focus adjustment function.

· 放射线区域监控（Radiation area monitoring）

确认治疗室内放射线区域监控设备的运作。

Confirm the operation of the indoor radiation monitoring equipment.

· 束流on表示（Beam on display）

确认使用束流时显示"照射中"字样。

Confirm that the word "irradiation" is displayed when using the beam.

· Snout冲突连锁（Snout conflict interlock）

确认Snout运作中的冲突连锁的运作情况。

Confirm the operation of the conflict interlock in the operation of the Snout.

· X射线装置冲突连锁（X-ray device conflict interlock）

确认X射线装置运作中的冲突连锁的运作情况。

Confirm the operation of the conflict interlock in the operation of the X-ray device.

· 患者用呼叫按钮（Patient call button）

按下患者用呼叫按钮确认运作情况。

Press the patient call button to confirm the operation.

26.2 每年的项目（Annual items）

· 急停开关的运作确认（Emergency stop switch operation confirmation）

确认急停开关结构、装置控制的各种连锁结构运作情况。

Confirm the operation of the interlock device of the emergency stop switch structure, device control.

第2节　trUpoint ARCH用户手册
User Manual of trUpoint ARCH

作者：李万国　张一贺　祁英　孟万斌　马霄云

本器械用于在立体定向放射治疗和立体定向放射手术期间大脑和头颈各部在体外放射治疗过程中的止动、定位以及重新定位。本器械还可用于图像采集时头部的止动和定位，以帮助制定采用计算机断层扫描技术（CT）及核磁共振成像（MRI）系统的治疗方案。

This instrument is used for the locking, immobilization and repositioning of the brain, head and neck during the stereotactic radiotherapy and stereotactic surgery. This instrument can also be used for the locking and immobilization of the head during image acquisition to help develop the treatment plan using computed tomography (CT) and MRI (magnetic resonance imaging) system.

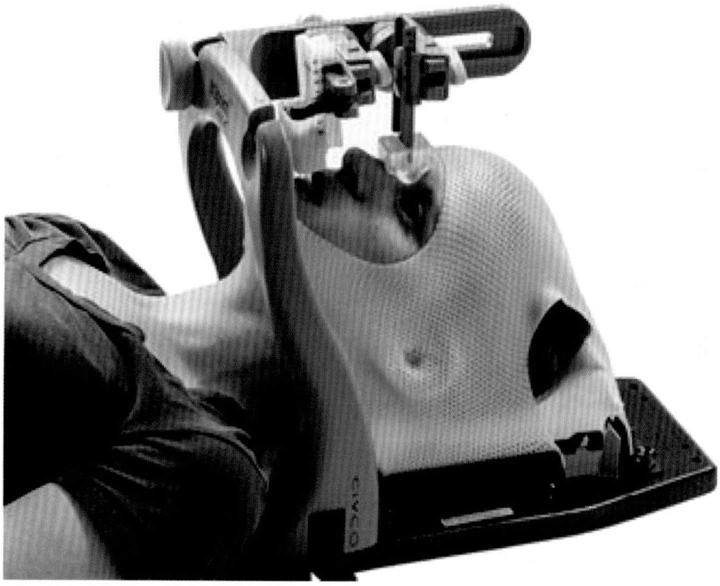

1 基板

(Base plate)

本器械，基本由PMMA基板本体和固定器具Lok-Bar组成。我们一般固定Lok-Bar于治疗床上，通过Lok-Bar的固定作用，再把基板固定于治疗床。

This instrument is composed of PMMA base plate body and fixed appliance Lok-Bar. We usually fix Lok-Bar on the treatment bed, and then fix the base plate to the treatment bed with the fixed function of Lok-Bar.

1.1 PMMA基板（PMMA Base Plate）

该器械基板由PMMA材料制成，为白色透明的头颈肩治疗板，设置有可固定于Lok-Bar的固定孔。使用时只需放置于已固定Lok-Bar的治疗床面上即可。

The base plate is made of PMMA(polymethyl methacrylate) materials, which is a white transparent head and shoulder treatment panel, with a hole that can be fixed to the Lok-Bar. When using, just place it on the treated bed surface with the fixed Lok-Bar.

1.2 Lok-Bar

该器械为碳纤维材料制成，符合碳离子治疗材料的要求。该器械不属于CIVCO公司trUpoint ARCH设备的出厂产品，也因治疗床的不同而不同，所以在使用时要选择治疗床配套的Lok-Bar，且在参数记录清单中一定要详细、准确地记录Lok-Bar的位置。因每个患者的位置不尽相同，故Lok-Bar的参数也会有所差异。所以精确地记录该器械的参数对于临床使用至关重要。

The instrument is made of carbon fiber and meets the requirements of carbon ion treatment materials. The device isn't CIVCO company trUpoint ARCH equipment. Products are also different due to different treatment bed. So when using, choose Lok-Bar which is assorted to the treatment bed, the location of the Lok-Bar should be recorded detailedly and accurately in the parameter list. The parameters of Lok-Bar vary depending on the location of each patient. So it is crucial for clinical use to accurately record the parameters of the device.

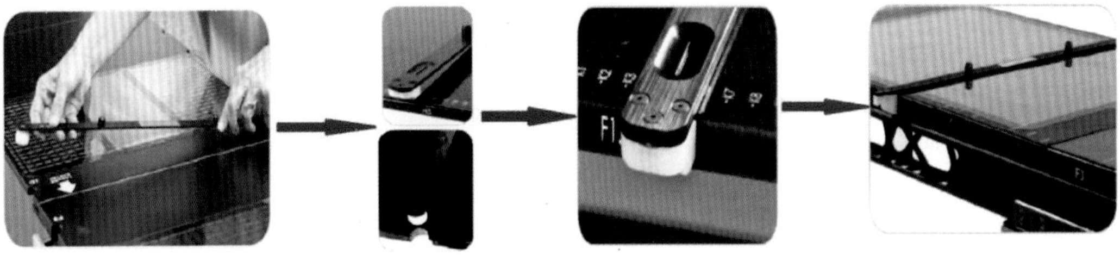

Lok-Bar	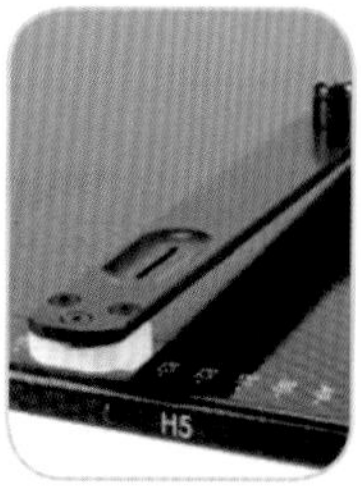	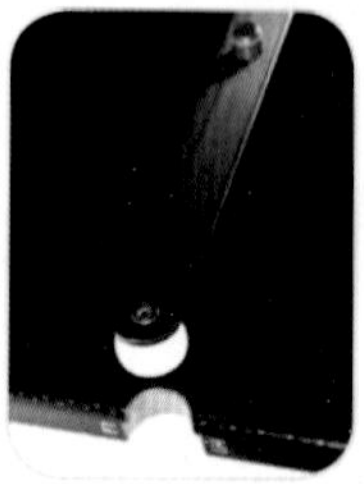
英 文 名	Prodigy™ 2	Interlock®
类　型	小凸球卡槽	大凹槽卡槽
间　距	7 cm	14 cm
适用范围	治疗室 CIVCO 床板	CT 室 SIEMENS 床板

2　船型头枕

(Individual head support)

船型头枕的使用相对较复杂，我们可以分解开来，按顺序依次完成。总体来讲可分为两个部分：(1) 压印泡沫枕体的固定；(2) 头枕热塑模的固定。

The use of the individual head support is relatively complicated. We can break it down and complete it in sequence. Generally speaking, it can be divided into two parts: (1) Fix of impression foam pillow; (2) fix of thermoplastic.

2.1　压印泡沫枕体 (Impression foam pillow)

泡沫枕体为橘黄色软泡沫塑性头枕，因为头部压力对头枕形成的形变不可恢复，所以可以记忆头部形状，更好地固定头部。该器械设置有若干卡扣，在 PMMA 基板上有完全适合头枕的固定卡槽。

Foam pillow is an orange soft foam plastic head pillow. Because the shape change caused by the head pressure can not restore, the pillow can remember the head shape and hold the head better. There are a number of clasps on the device and there are anchor card slots fit for the headrest on the PMMA substrate.

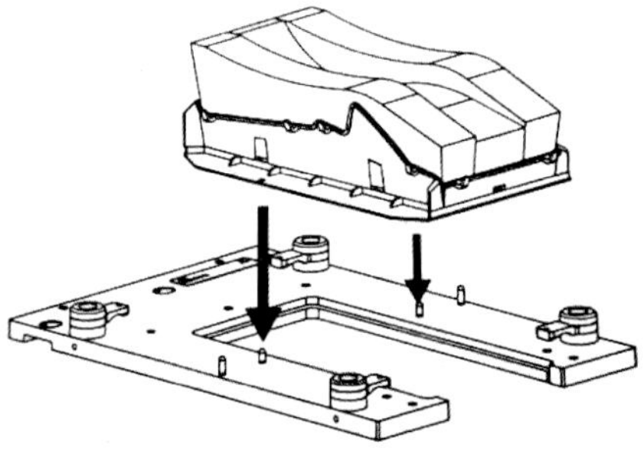

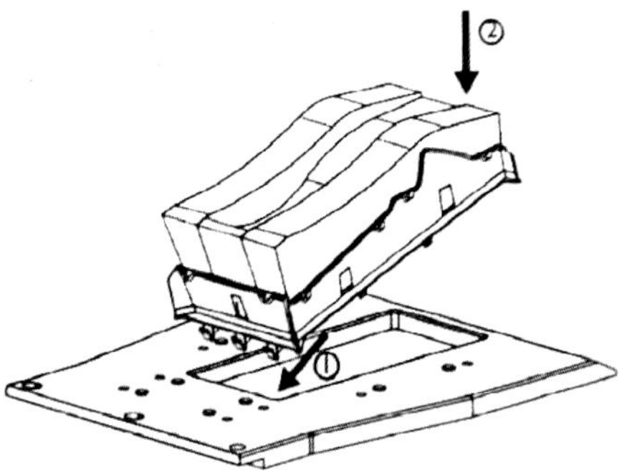

2.2 头枕热塑模（Thermoplastic）

该器械的使用方法与普通放射治疗定位时所用的热塑膜的使用方法基本相同，我们可参考其中的经验方法。不同的且复杂的地方就在于头枕热塑模卡扣的设置。卡扣与压印泡沫枕体上的挂钩配套使用，可使热塑模固定于压印泡沫枕体上，形成完整的可供使用的船型头枕。

The method of using the apparatus is basically the same as the thermoplastic used in the localization of conventional radiotherapy. We can refer to the empirical method. Different and complicated place lies in the headrest thermal mold card settings. Card buckle linked to stamping on foam pillow body, can make the hot mold be fixed on the embossing foam pillow body, form a complete ship type head that can be used.

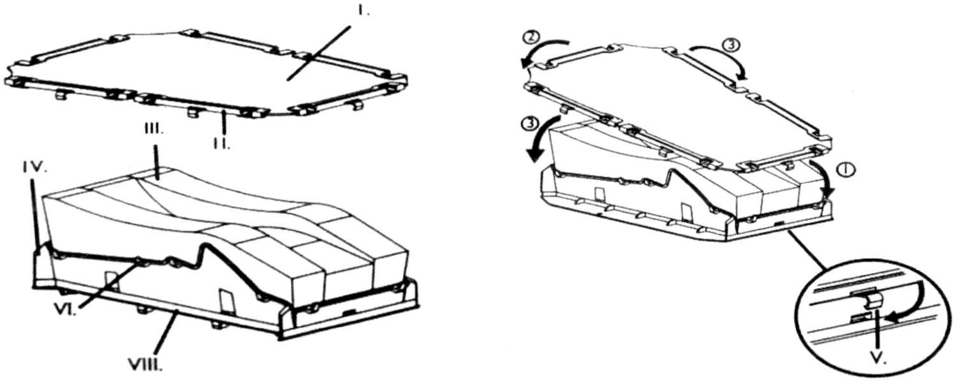

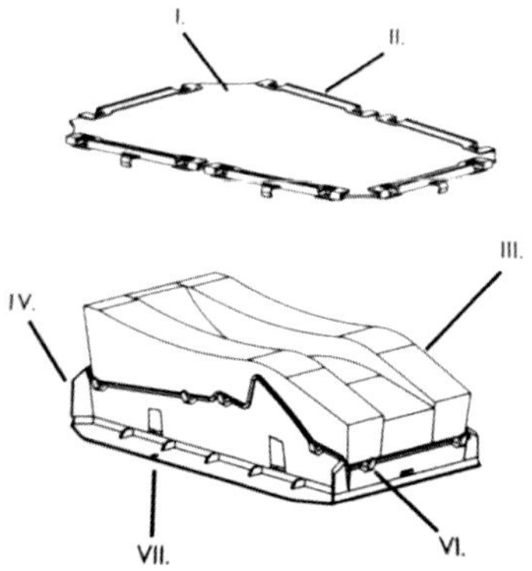

Ⅰ热塑膜　Ⅱ热塑膜外形　Ⅲ 压印泡沫　Ⅳ 锁夹　Ⅴ 挂钩　Ⅵ 枕体基座

Ⅰ Thermoplastic　Ⅱ Profile　Ⅲ Impression Foam　Ⅳ Holder　Ⅴ Hook Ⅵ Pillow Base Plate

综上所述，船型头枕的制作流程可总结如下：

（1）向水箱中注入足以淹没热塑膜厚度的水，加热至75 ℃。

（2）将压印泡沫、固定器和基座组件按图示放在定位装置上。

（3）在不压缩泡沫的情况下，对患者预定位，以使患者的头部枕在头部支架所需的位置。

（4）将头枕热塑模放在水箱中1分钟左右时间，从水箱中取出时查看热塑膜有无大面积的硬块存在，一般在水量、水温和时间都满足要求的情况下热塑模软硬适中即可使用。切不可长时间置于水箱中。

（5）用干毛巾除去热塑模材料上多余的水分。

（6）按图示，将热塑模和外形连接到固定器上，固定时务必注意热塑膜的光面在里、织物面在外。

（7）按照预定位时的经验，将患者的头部固定在船型头枕上。

（8）向患者的前额施加一定的压力，确保患者的后脑部分镶嵌到船型头枕里，以达到所需的位置。

（9）让热塑膜冷却5～10分钟，放下患者即可。

The work flow of how to make the pillow is as follows:

（1）Pump sufficient water into the tank which is more drawn the thermoplastic, heat the water to 75 ℃.

（2）Place impression foam, holder and base assembly on positioning device as shown.

（3）Preposition patient without compressing foam so head will rest in desired location on head support.

（4）Place thermoplastic in water bath for 1 minute. Remove thermoplastic from water bath and check whether there are extensive nuggets on the thermoplastic. It can be used if it is neither hard nor soft as while as the volume and temperature of the water and the time meet the demand. No being in the tank for a long time!

（5）Remove excess water from thermoplastic.

（6）Attach thermoplastic and profiles to holder as shown, ensure the smooth surface of the thermoplastic inside and the fabric surface outside.

（7）Place patient's head on head support depending on the experience of preposition.

（8）Press patient into head support by placing pressure on forehead and chin to achieve desired position.

（9）Cool thermoplastic for 5–10 minutes and lay the patient.

警告：

（1）整个设置及治疗期间，本器械仅限使用于一名患者。切勿使用于其他患者，以免传染疾病，为治疗带来不必要的麻烦。

（2）压印泡沫在使用前无过度的形变。

（3）对于该器械的废弃处理，务必遵守我院制定的感染控制政策。

（4）工作人员务必佩戴一次性口罩和一次性手套，以避免患者、同事和本人受感染。

WARNING:

(1) During the whole setting and treatment, this instrument is restricted to only one patient. Do not use it in other patients, so as not to spread the disease and bring unnecessary trouble to the treatment.

(2) The pressure printing foam has no excessive deformation before use.

(3) For the disposal of this instrument, it is important to follow the infection control policy established by our hospital.

(4) Staff must wear disposable masks and disposable gloves to avoid infection with patients, colleagues and themselves.

3 热塑膜面罩

(Thermoplastic mask)

热塑膜面罩的制作对于头部的固定是非常重要的，因为热塑膜面罩会把整个头部完全包在面罩内，所以在制作面罩之前咬合托盘必须事先制作完成，且不可在热塑膜面罩制作完之后再去完成咬合托盘，以免对热塑膜面罩的使用造成一定的影响。所以对于热塑膜面罩我们分两部分去完成：(1) 咬合托盘；(2) 热塑膜面罩。

Thermoplastic film mask making is very important for the head fix. Because thermoplastic film mask would make the whole head in the mask, before making mask bite cup must be completed in advance, and never be made after thermoplastic film mask making, in order to avoid affecting the use of thermoplastic film mask. So for the thermoplastic mask is completed in two steps: (1)bite cup; (2)thermoplastic mask.

3.1 咬合托盘 (Bite cup)

如图，咬合托盘的制作可分为三步：

(1) 根据病人自身的情况，选择合适的咬合托盘。可供选择的咬合托盘型号有C6901、C6902、C6903、C6904、C6905，共五种尺寸。我们要根据病人上颌骨的大小，选择合适的咬合托盘尺寸。

(2) 用牙胶枪在咬合托盘的凹槽内打入适量的牙胶，大约有凹槽体积的三分之二为宜。

(3) 牙胶填充完毕后，快速将咬合托盘置入患者的口中，务必要保证托盘的凹槽向上、患者的上颚牙齿完全陷入咬合托盘凹槽的牙胶中，让病人保持最舒适的口型，待三分钟左右的时间即可将已经成型的咬合托盘取出。

Making the bite cup can be divided into three steps as follows:

(1) According to a patient's own condition, select the appropriate bite cup. Available cup types include C6901, C6902, C6903, C6904, C6905, a total of five dimensions. We should

choose the appropriate bite cup size according to the size of the patient's upper jaw.

(2) The glue gun is used to put tooth gum in the grooves of the bit cup and the proper amount of the gums is about two-thirds of the volume of the grooves.

(3) After the tooth gum being filled, put the bit cup into the mouth of the patient quickly. Be sure that the grooves of the bit cup is upward and the patient's upper jaw teeth in the gum of the grooves of the bit cup completely. Keep the patient's mouth the most comfortable state. The molding bit cup can be trayed out for about 3 minutes.

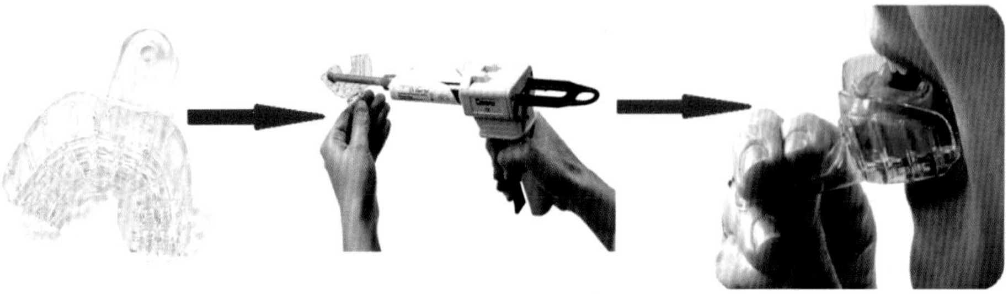

警告:

(1) 整个制作及治疗期间，本器械仅限使用于一名患者。禁止使用于其他患者，以免传染疾病，为治疗带来不必要的麻烦。

(2) 在整个治疗期间要严格保证咬合托盘的卫生质量，且不可随意乱放，造成不必要的污染。

(3) 对于该器械的废弃处理，务必遵守我院制定的感染控制政策。

(4) 工作人员务必佩戴一次性口罩和一次性手套，以避免人为的因素污染咬合托盘。

WARNING:

(1) During the whole setting and treatment, this instrument is restricted to only one patient. Do not use it in other patients, so as not to spread the disease and bring unnecessary trouble to the treatment.

(2) During the whole treatment, it is necessary to ensure the hygienic quality of the bite cup, and not randomly placed, so as not to cause unnecessary pollution.

(3) For the disposal of this instrument, it is important to follow the infection control policy established by our hospital.

(4) Staff must wear disposable masks and disposable gloves to avoid infection with patients, colleagues and themselves.

3.2 热塑膜面罩（Thermoplastic film mask）

trUpoint ARCH热塑膜面罩（Posicast-Lite , Head-Only and H, N & S）是配合ARCH使用的特制面罩，较传统的热塑膜面罩而言，该热塑膜面罩在与患者的接触一侧有一种柔软的聚氨酯涂料，使患者更加舒适；而另一边则有光滑的喷漆，以方便在面罩上做出治疗标记。它的制作技术要求与传统的热塑膜制作技术要求基本相同。可总结如下：

TrUpoint ARCH thermoplastic film mask (Posicast-Lite, Head-Only the and H, N and S) is a specialty mask used with the ARCH. Compared with the traditional thermoplastic film, the thermoplastic film mask in contact with the patient's side there is a kind of soft polyurethane coating, to make patients more comfortable. On the other side, there is a smooth spray paint to facilitate the treatment of the mask. The technical requirements of its production are similar to that of traditional thermal plastic film production. It can be summarized as follows:

Posicast-Lite技术要求参数				
尺寸(mm)	加热水温	加热时间	塑型时间	冷却时间
299 L × 372 W × 27 T	70 ℃	1 min	1 min 15 sec	8 min 45 sec

(1) 取出我们专用的trUpoint热塑膜置于水温为70℃的水箱中，加热时间以1 min为宜，时间过长或过短都会对热塑膜的正常使用有较大的影响。

(2) 取出已加热好的热塑膜，用毛巾轻触，除去多余的水分。

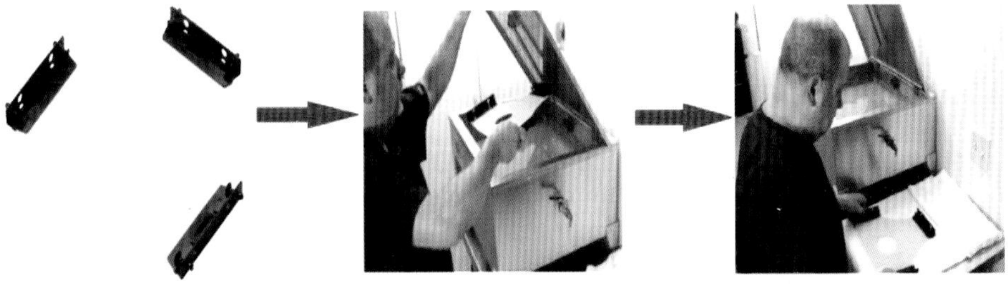

(3) 按照下图的方式，进行热塑膜的制作。在整个的制作过程要保证患者没有过度的移动。

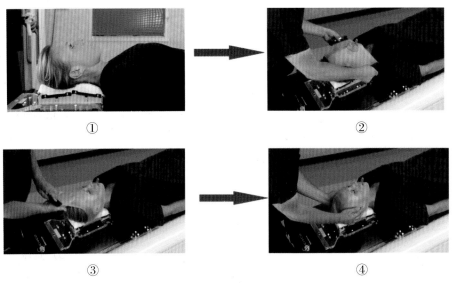

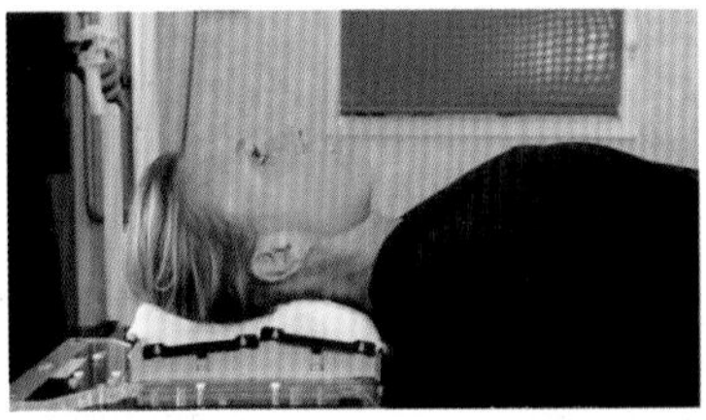

①

②

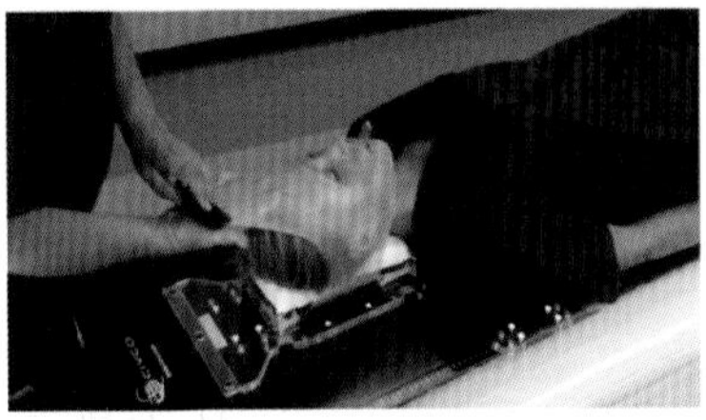

③

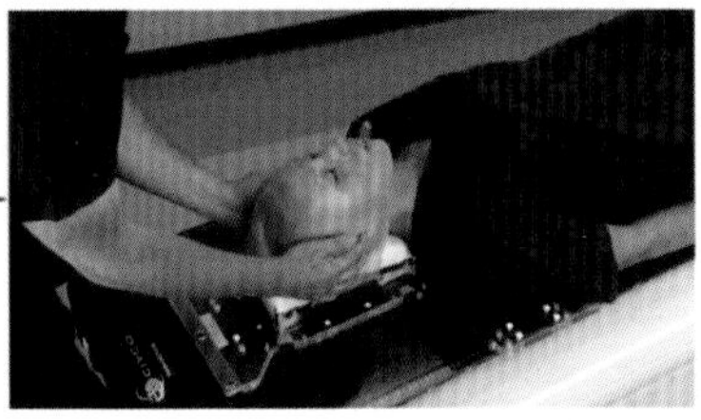

④

（4）待热塑膜塑型完成后，参考技术标准，冷却时间为 8 min 45 s。正常情况下，一般都让患者静坐 10 min 为宜。在冷却的过程中要严密观察患者的头部，叮嘱患者切勿移动头部，以免对精确地塑型造成大的影响。如果发现患者的移动幅度较大，或者热塑膜的塑型没有达到预期效果，应立即将面罩取下并置于水箱中，重复以上操作，进行患者再定位。

（1）Take out our dedicated trUpoint thermoplastic film in the water tank when the water temperature is 70 ℃, the heating time is 1 min advisable, too long or too short time for the normal use of thermoplastic film have a great influence.

（2）Remove the heated plastic film that has been heated and gently touch it with a towel to remove excess water.

（3）Make the thermal plastic film according to the picture. Be sure that the patient dosn't move excessively during the whole making process.

（4）After the shaping of thermoplastic film was completed, according to the reference technology standard, the cooling time is 8 min 45 s. Normally, it is advisable for patients to sit for 10 min. In the process of cooling, the patient's head should be closely monitored, and the patient should not move the head to avoid affecting the accuracy of the shaping. If it is found that the patient's movements are larger, or thermoplastic film shape did not achieve the desired effect, the mask will be immediately removed and put in the tank, repeat the above operation, replace the patient.

警告：

参考压印泡沫头枕的警告注意事项。

WARNING:

Refer to the warning notes for impression foam pillow.

4 trUpoint

trUpoint 的设置在头部肿瘤患者的体位固定中是复杂的，也是最后的一项工作，上面需要调节的参数极多，在使用之前，我们一定要花时间去熟悉 ARCH 的所有功能的使用，以便在后面的使用中提高效率。

TrUpoint settings is complex in the immobilization of head tumor patients and is the last work. There are many parameters to adjust. Before use it, we must take time to be familiar with the use of all functions of the ARCH, in order to improve efficiency in the use of in the rear.

我们可按照下面图示的方法去熟悉该设备的所有操作：

The basic operation of trUpoint is shown as the following:

（1）松开框架臂上的大旋钮，将框架臂旋转到反方向，并拧紧旋钮固定好。

Loosen large knob on frame arm. Rotate frame arm into opposite orientation and tighten knob to secure.

（2）松开鼻根组件臂上的中旋钮，将组件旋转到180°，并拧紧旋钮固定好。

Loosen medium knob on nasion assembly arm. Rotate assembly 180° and tighten knob to secure.

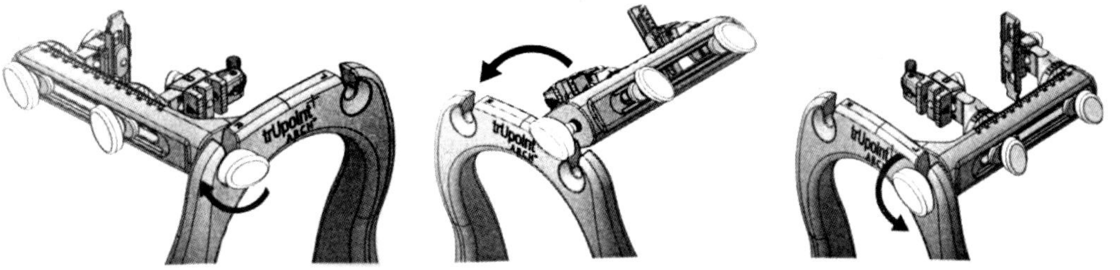

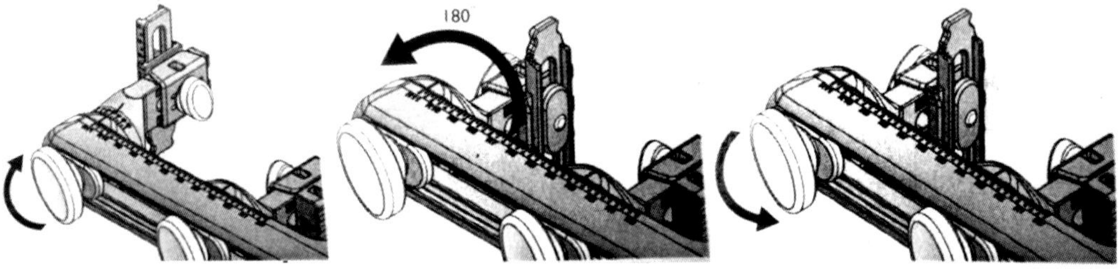

（3）松开咬合组件臂上的中旋钮，将组件旋转180°，并拧紧旋钮固定好。

Loosen medium knob on bite assembly arm. Rotate assembly 180° and tighten knob to secure.

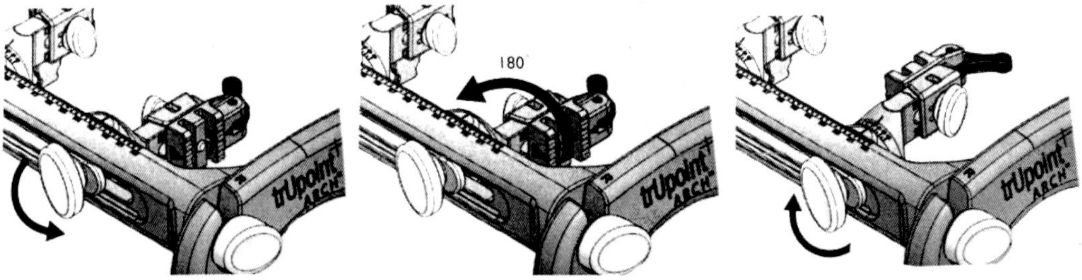

（4）松开鼻根组件上的小旋钮，将组件滑出组件臂，使用组件臂上侧的小旋钮重新装上组件，并拧紧旋钮固定好。

Loosen small knob on nasion assembly to slide assembly off arm. Replace assembly with small knob on superior side of arm and tighten knob to secure.

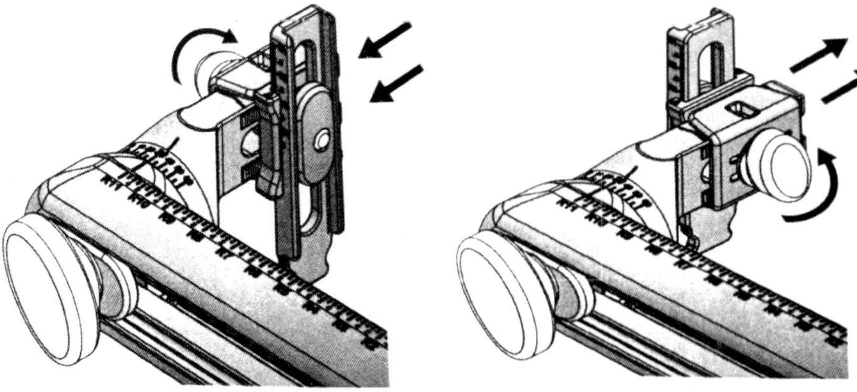

（5）松开咬合组件上的小旋钮，将组件滑出组件臂，使用组件臂上侧的小旋钮重新装上组件，并拧紧旋钮固定好。

Loosen small knob on bite assembly to slide assembly off arm. Replace assembly with small knob on superior side of arm and tighten knob to secure.

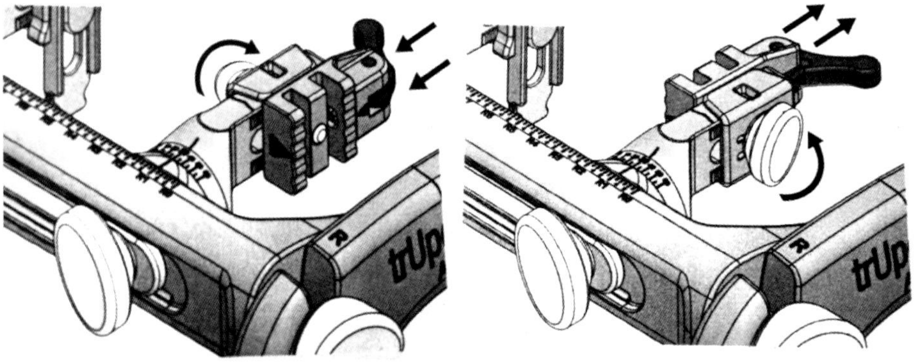

（6）确保咬合组件上的黑色拉杆未锁定，将咬合杯放在咬合组件中，锁紧黑色拉杆以固定好。

Ensure black lever on bite assembly is unlocked. Place bite cup in bite assembly and lock black lever to secure.

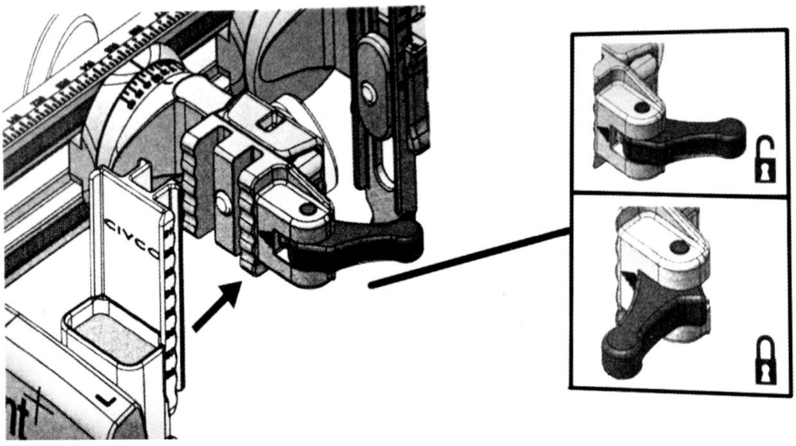

4.1 鼻根组件初始设置（Initial setup of nasion systems）

鼻根组件也是CIVCO公司特殊设计的配套ARCH使用的组件，是呈白色半透明状、质软的方形部件，只为在鼻根部位压住患者，以固定患者的头部。该部件的使用也较简单，我们可参考下图去完成设置。

Nasion systems component is also special designed by CIVCO company to support the use of the ARCH components, which is a white translucent, soft square part, just for pressing patients in nasal root to fix the patient's head. The use of the component is also simpler, and we can refer to the following figure to complete the setup.

（1）将鼻根垫连接到鼻根杆。

Attach nasion cushion to nasion stem.

（2）将鼻根组件放到最高位置并拧紧小旋钮。

Position nasion assembly in the highest position and tighten small knob.

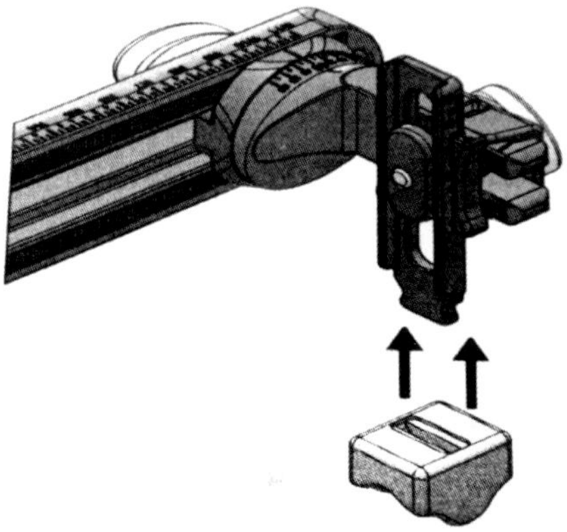

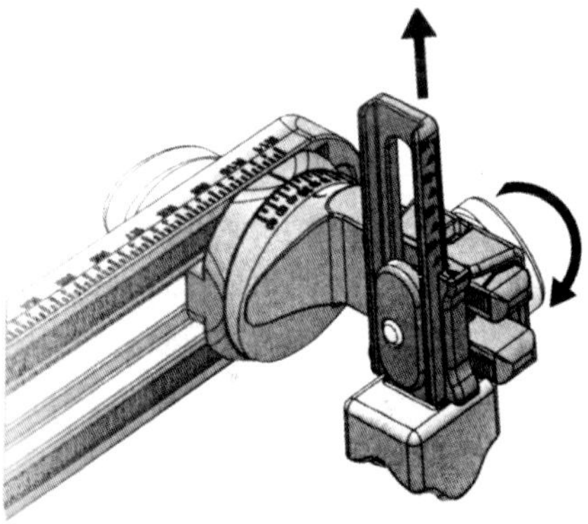

（3）松开组件臂上的中旋钮，并将其从弓形架中滑出，拧紧旋钮固定好。

Loosen medium knobs on assembly arm and slide away from arch. Tighten knobs to secure.

（4）将基座固定锁保持在完全向上的位置，并通过将定位插销插入颈部位置的孔中，将trUpoint ARCH安装到基板。

Hold base locks in full upward position and attach trUpoint ARCH to base plate by inserting locating pins into holes at the neck position.

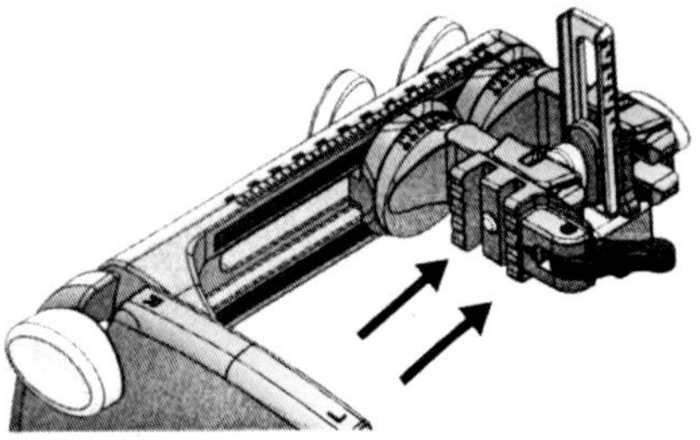

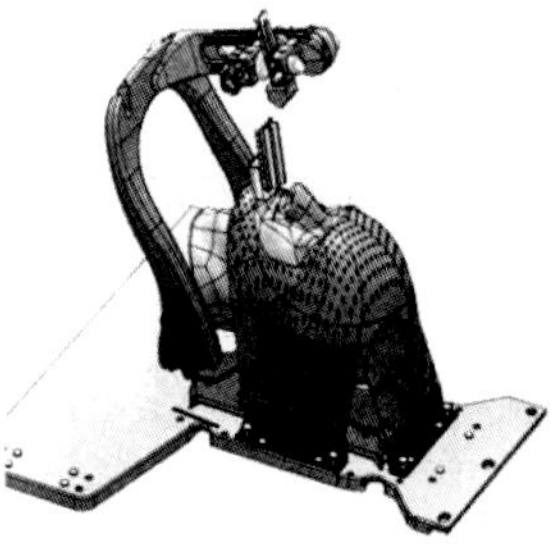

（5）将基座固定锁向下推以固定好。

Push base locks downward to secure.

4.2 咬合杯初始设置（Initial setup of bite cup）

咬合器组件的设置极为复杂，按照之前的方法，我们提前熟悉咬合器组件的各项相关功能，例如：各旋钮的功能、横向纵向移动的实现等。只要熟练掌握了该组件各项功能的使用，我们可按照下图所示的方法实现咬合组件的设置：

The set of bite cup components is very complex, in accordance with the previous methods, we are familiar with all the related functions of clutch components in advance, such as: the function of each knob, the realization of the transverse and longitudinal movement, etc. As long as the use of various functions of this component is mastered, we can implement the setting of occlusion components according to the method shown below:

（1）解锁咬合组件上的黑色拉杆，首次设置前，松开咬合组件上的小旋钮和咬合组件臂上的中旋钮。

Unlock black lever on bite assembly. Loosen small knob on bite assembly and medium knob on bite assembly arm prior to initial set-up.

（2）将咬合托盘放入患者口中，将咬合杯直接持放在咬合托盘杆上方，朝咬合杯方向滑动咬合组件，获得所需的直线位置，然后调整咬合组件臂到所需的角度，拧紧咬合组件上的小旋钮和组件臂上的中旋钮以固定好。

With bite tray in patient' s mouth, hole bite cup directly over bite tray stem. Slide bite assembly arm toward bite cup to obtain desired linear position and adjust bite assembly arm to desired angle. Tighten small knob on bite assembly and medium knob on assembly arm to secure.

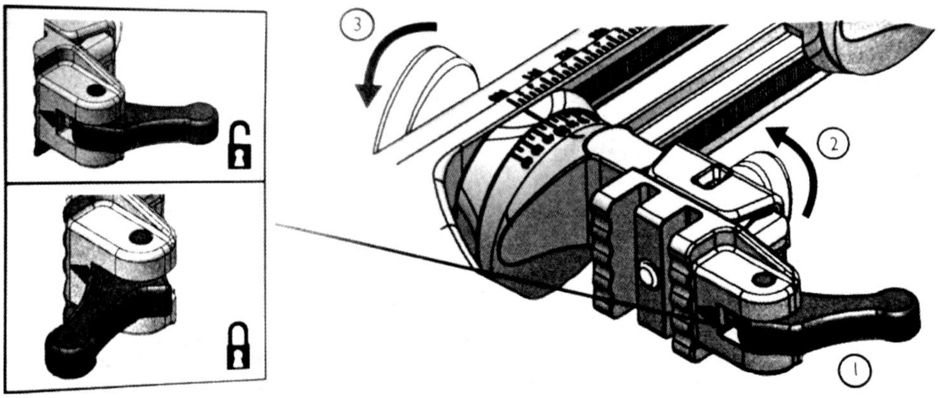

（3）调整咬合杯到所需的垂直位置，并锁住咬合组件上的黑色拉杆以固定好。

Adjust bite cup to desired vertical position and lock black lever on bite assembly to secure.

警告：

（1）将咬合杯放在离患者嘴唇尽可能近但不能接触的位置上。

（2）确保从咬合杯的顶部两个孔中可以看见咬合托盘杆的弓形结构。

WARNING:

（1）Put bite cup as close to patient's lips as possible without touching.

（2）Ensure arch of bite tray stem is visible in the top two holes of bite cup.

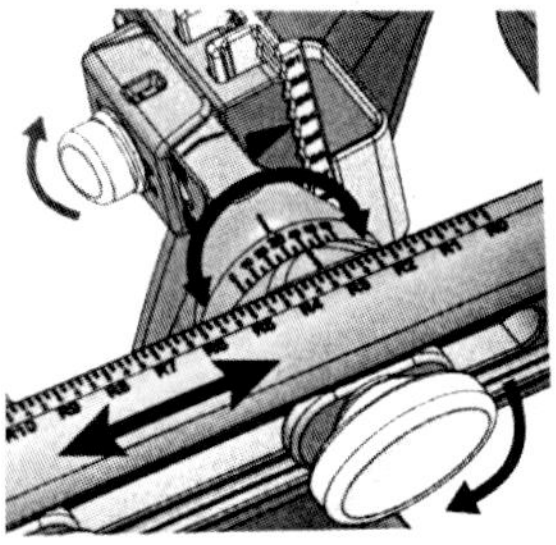

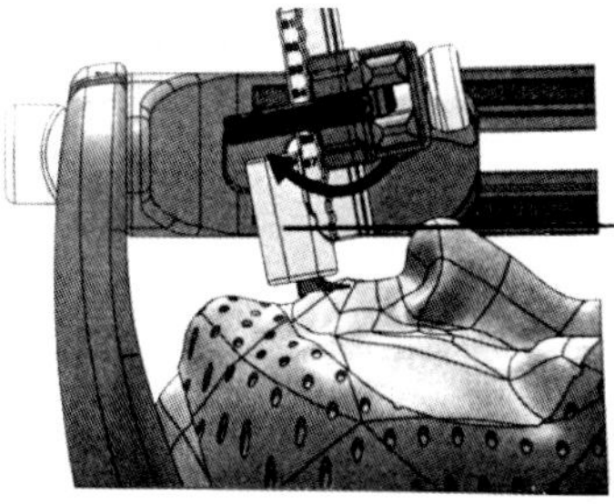

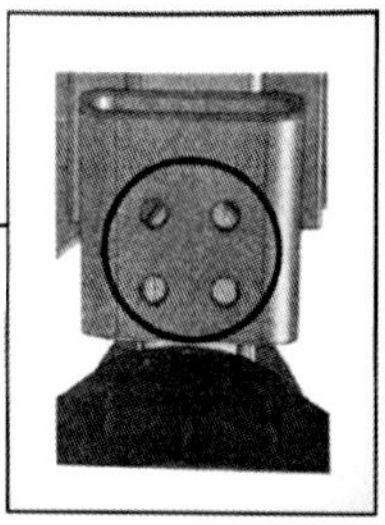

（4）将牙胶注入咬合托盘杆周围的咬合杯，确保牙胶完全填满咬合杯底部，等待牙胶完全硬化。

Insert putty into bite cup around bite tray stem. Ensure putty fills the bite cup completely. Allow putty to fully harden.

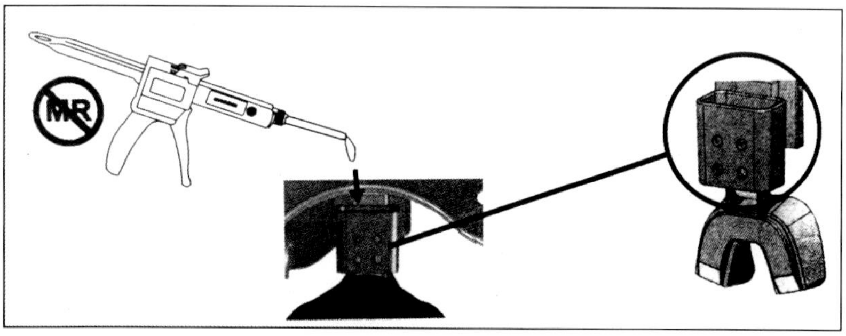

4.3　调节咬合组件（Adjusting bite assembly）

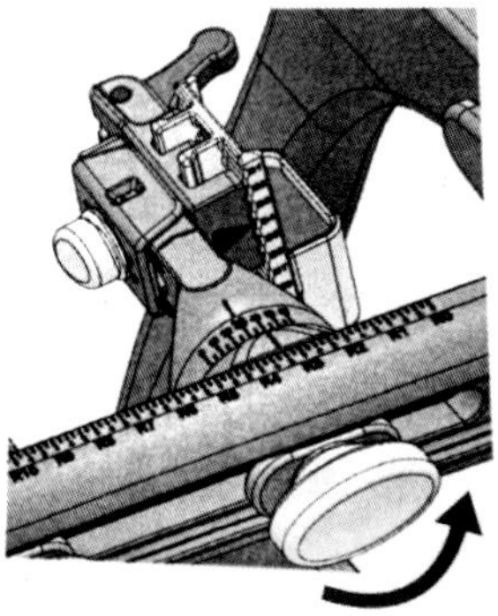

松开咬合组件臂上的中旋钮
Loosen medium knobs on bite assembly arm

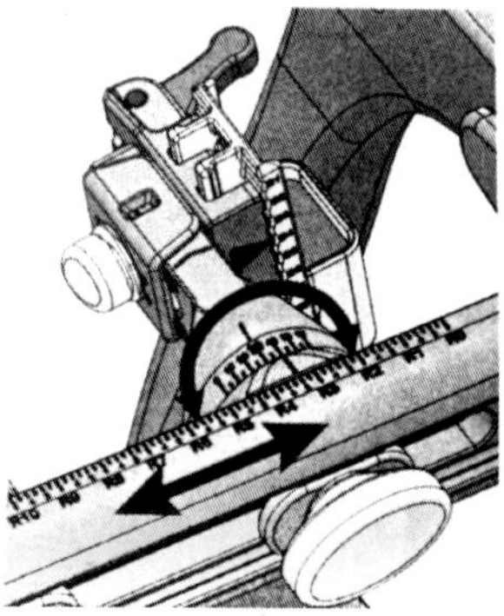

将组件调整到所需角度，并滑到所需的直线位置
Adjust the assembly to the desired angle, and slide it to the desired linear position

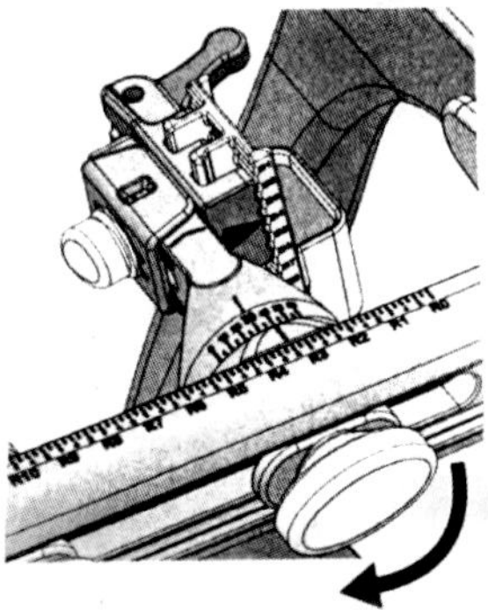

拧紧中旋钮以固定好
Tighten medium knobs to secure

4.4 调节咬合杯（Adjusting bite cup）

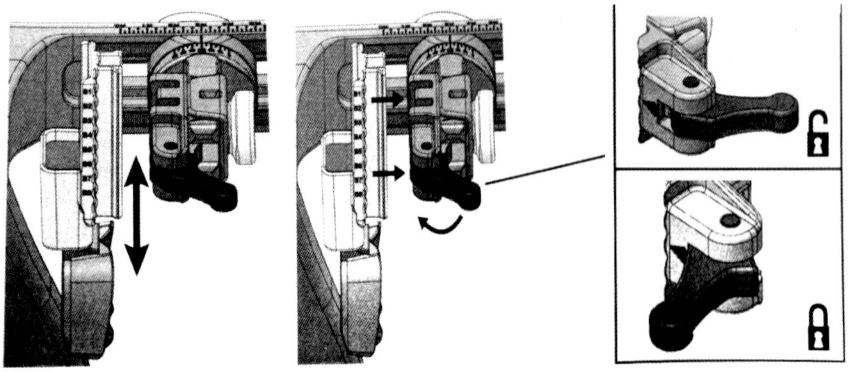

将咬合杯滑到适当的垂直位置
Slide bite cup to appropriate vertical position

将咬合杯放在咬合组件中，锁紧黑色拉杆以固定好
Place bite cup in bite assembly and lock black lever to secure

4.5 调节鼻根组件（Adjusting nasion assembly）

（1）松开鼻根组件上的小旋钮。

Loosen small knob on nasion assembly.

（2）将鼻根垫放在患者的鼻梁接合处的下部弓上，最后进行垂直调节，拧紧以固定好。

Put nasion cushion at lower arch of patient' s nose bridge junction. Make vertical adjustment at last. Tighten small knob to secure.

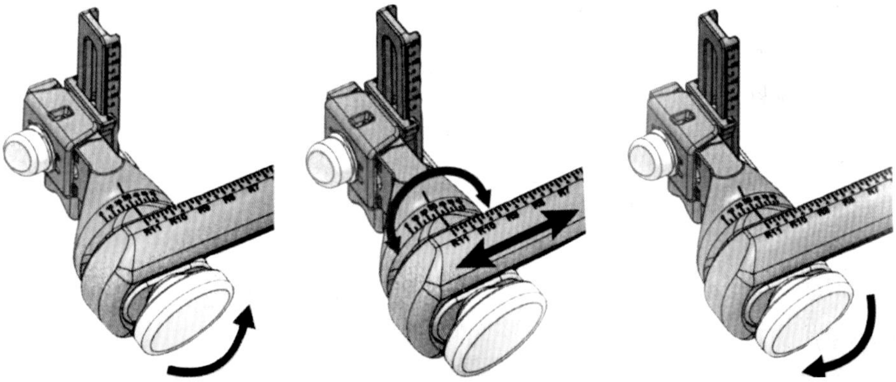

松开鼻根组件臂上的中旋钮
Loosen medium knobs on nasion assembly arm

将组件调整到所需角度，并滑到所需的直线位置
Adjust the nasion assembly to desired angle, and slide to desired linear position

拧紧中旋钮以固定好
Tighten medium knobs to secure

警告：

鼻根部件也是患者特有的组件，请务必参照压印泡沫头枕、咬合杯等一次性使用组件的注意事项。

The nasion assembly is also a special component for the patient, please be sure to use the attention of the foam head pillow, bite cup, etc.

4.6 ARCH参数记录单（ARCH Setup Sheet）

在整个trUpoint ARCH设置及制作完成后，务必将该患者所使用的trUpoint ARCH所有的参数进行详细的记录。我们已经设计好相应的参数记录表（后附），请按照该参数记录表详细记录。

After the entire trUpoint ARCH setup and production are completed, it is important to keep a detailed record of all the parameters used for the patient in trUpoint ARCH. We have designed the corresponding parameter record form (attached). Please record it in detail according to this parameter record.

4.7 卸下trUpoint ARCH（Removing trUpoint ARCH）

移除trUpoint ARCH前，确保填妥设置单以记录患者有关的设置参数。

Ensure setup sheet is complete to record patient settings prior to removing trUpoint ARCH.

（1）解锁咬合组件上的黑色拉杆，解开咬合杯。

Unlock black lever on bite assembly to release bite cup.

（2）必要时，松开中旋钮，将咬合组件滑离咬合杯。

Loosen medium knob and slide bite assembly away from bite cup, if necessary.

（3）向上提起基座固定锁，将trUpoint ARCH从基板中卸下。

Lift base locks upward and remove trUpoint ARCH from base plate.

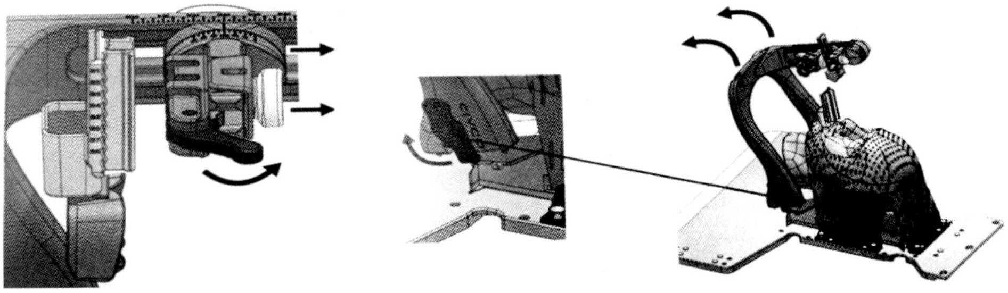

至此，trUpoint ARCH所有的制作就圆满完成了，我们现在要做的就是保存好患者信息记录单、取下trUpoint ARCH组件、叮嘱患者进行后续的治疗。

So far, trUpoint ARCH has been completed successfully, and what we need to do now is to save the patient's information sheet, to remove the trUpoint ARCH component, and to instruct the patient to follow up the treatment.

附件：CIVCO设置参数记录单（ARCH Sheet）

CIVCO 设置参数记录单
trUpoint ARCH

trUpoint ARCH™

姓名：________________ 日期：________________
备注：____

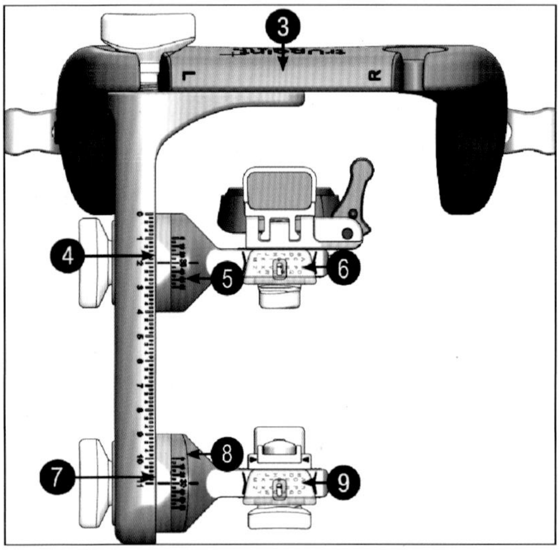

1. 基板类型：
2. 船型头枕：
3. 弓形架位置：
R L
4. 咬合器组件纵向位置:
0|2|4| 2|2|4| 3|2|4| 4|2|4| 5|2|4| 6|2|4|
6|2|4| 7|2|4| 8|2|4| 9|2|4| 10|2|4| 11|2|4|
5. 咬合器组件旋转位置
0 5 10 15 20 25 30 35 40 45 50 55 60
6. 咬合器组件横向位置
A B C D E F G H I J K L M N
O P Q R S T U V W X Y Z
7. 鼻根组件纵向位置
0|2|4| 2|2|4| 3|2|4| 4|2|4| 5|2|4| 6|2|4|
6|2|4| 7|2|4| 8|2|4| 9|2|4| 10|2|4| 11|2|4|

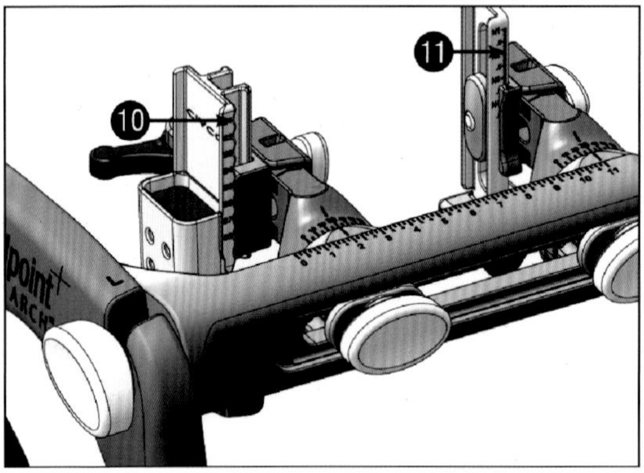

8. 鼻根组件旋转位置
0 5 10 15 20 25 30 35 40 45 50 55 60
9. 鼻根组件横向位置
A B C D E F G H I J K L M N
O P Q R S T U V W X Y Z
10. 咬合器组件垂直位置
B1 B2 B3 B4 B5 B6 B7 B8
11. 鼻根组件垂直位置
N1 ||||. 5 |||| N2 ||||. 5 ||||
N3 ||||. 5 |||| N4 ||||. 5 ||||

操作技师：
日　　期：

第3节　头颈部肿瘤患者体位固定标准操作流程
Standard Operating Procedure for the Immobilization of Head and Neck Tumor Patients

作者：李万国　张一贺　祁英　孟万斌　马霄云

头颈部肿瘤患者体位固定是所有体位固定中最为复杂的一种，但根据我们光子以及日本、德国重离子及质子体位固定的经验，我们也可以采用热塑膜加头枕的固定方式来实现。下面就详细阐述头颈肩部位肿瘤患者体位固定的标准操作流程。

Immobilization of head and neck tumor patients is one of the most complex kind of immobilization. But according to our photon and Japan, Germany heavy ion and proton immobilization experience, we can also adopt thermoplastic film head fixed way to implement. The standard operating procedure of the immobilization of head, neck and shoulder tumor patients is described in detail below.

1　底板（又名延伸板）固定
(Basic Plate Fixed)

1.1　Lok-Bar

底板的固定，首先由固定底板的固定条Lok-Bar开始。这是专用于SBRT板上的一种锁定条，由碳纤维材料制成，符合碳离子治疗的材料要求。

The base plate is fixed, starting with a fixed strip of fixed Bar Lok-Bar. This is a kind of locking bar dedicated to SBRT, made of carbon fiber material, which meets the material requirements of carbon ion therapy.

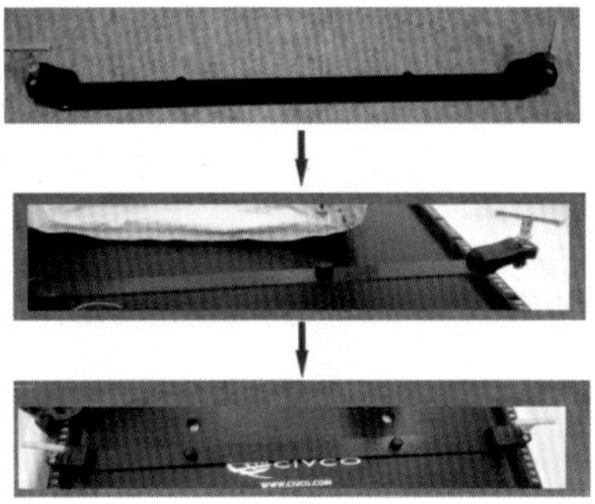

1.2 底板固定（Basic Plate Fixed）

对于目前的底板，我们通常采用如图所示的底板固定方式，但很多情况下出于稳定性的考虑，除了用Lok-Bar来固定，我们还会加一条带子，把底板绑在治疗床上。

For the base plate, we usually adopt bottom fixed way as shown. But in many cases, for the sake of the stability, in addition to use Lok - Bar to fixed, we will add a strap to tie plate in the treatment bed.

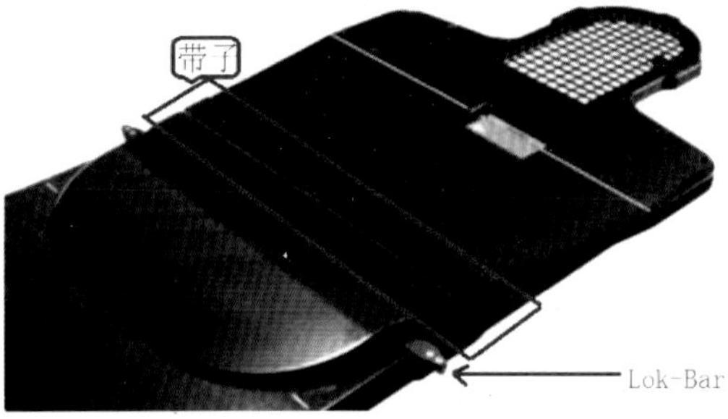

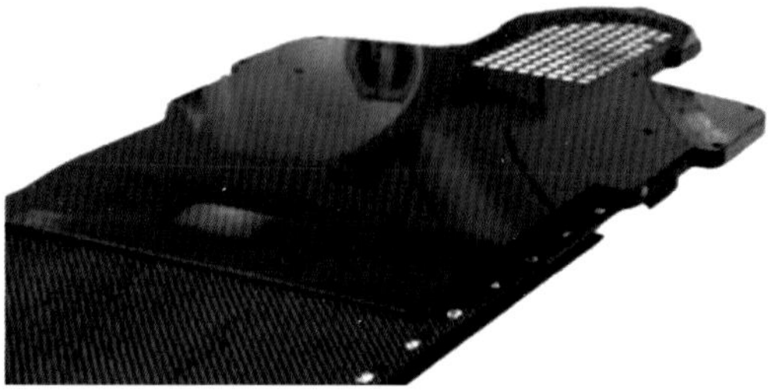

2 头枕制作 (Pillow Making)

此底板上可用的头枕种类很多，我们可根据患者的实际情况选择不同的头枕。

There are many kinds of head pillow available on this base plate. We can choose different pillow according to the actual situation of patients.

有关头枕的制作流程，我们可参考灰袋子以及咬合器头枕的制作流程。在头枕制作完成后，请务必将患者的信息在头枕上用标签标明，以免弄混患者信息，为后期的治疗带来不必要的麻烦。

For the production of the pillow, we can refer to the production process of the gray bag and the pillow of the bite block. After the pillow making is finished, please be sure to label the patient' s information on the pillow, so as not to confuse the patient information, and cause unnecessary trouble during the later treatment.

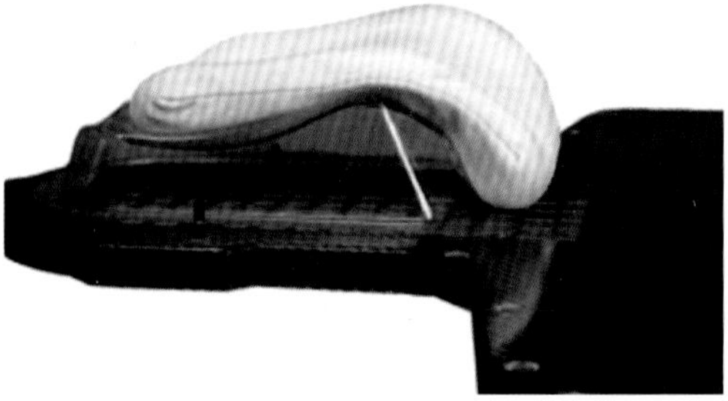

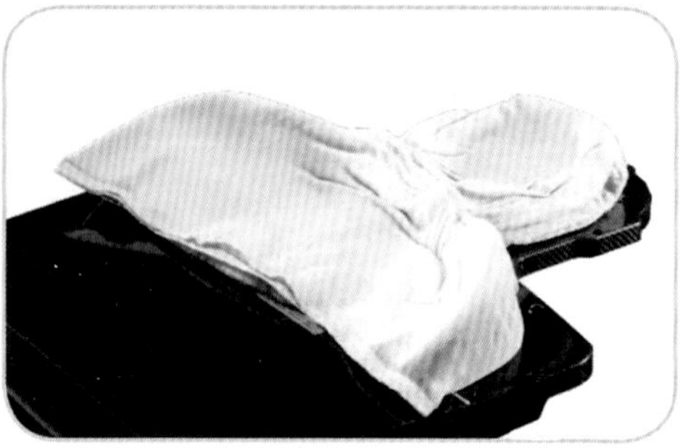

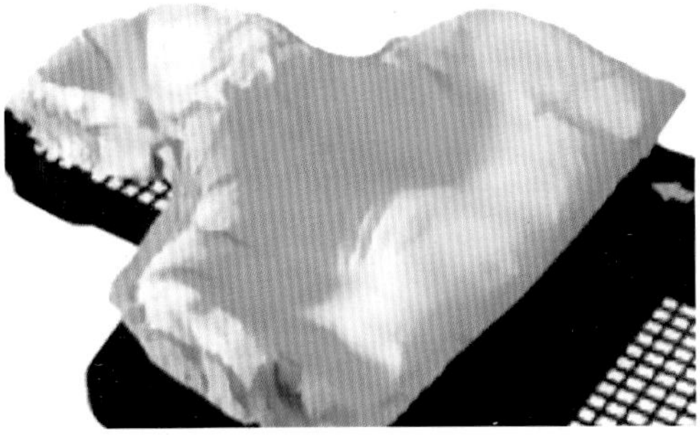
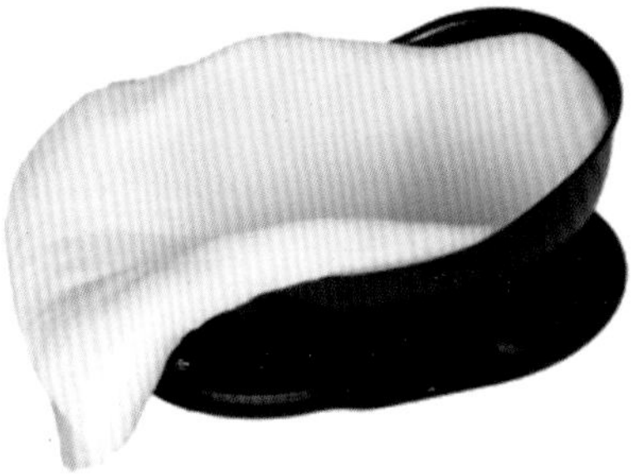

3 患者体位确认
(Patient Position Confirmation)

如图所示，我们采用患者仰卧位，双手平放于体侧，双眼直视上方，尽量使患者保持最舒适的躺姿，且该姿势能保持相对较长的时间，以便于技师进行固定膜具制作。

As shown, we adopt the patient supine, hands flat on body side, his eyes looking straight at the top to keep patients with the most comfortable lying posture as far as possible, and the position can maintain a relatively long time, so that the technicians can make the fixing mask.

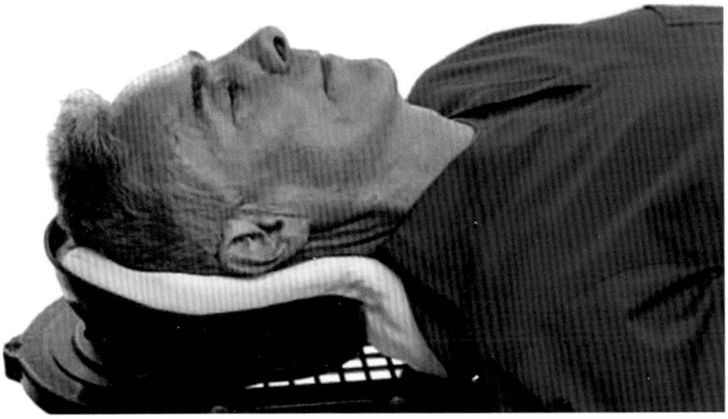

4 热塑膜制作
(Thermoplastic Mask Making)

热塑膜的种类也千差万别，也要根据患者的实际情况去选择不同的热塑膜。

The types of thermoplastic masks vary widely and different thermoplastic masks are selected according to the patient's actual situation.

选择好合适的热塑膜之后，把该热塑膜放进水箱，我们可根据如表所示的数据进行操作，以保证最高效、最合理地使用，达到最好的效果。

Choose suitable thermoplastic mask. Put the thermoplastic mask in the water tank. We can ensure the most efficient and reasonable use according to the data, as shown in the table, to achieve the best effect.

热塑膜技术要求参数				
尺寸(mm)	加热水温	加热时间	塑型时间	冷却时间
299 L × 372 W × 27 T	70 ℃	1 min	1 min15 sec	8 min45 sec

接下来，我们可用如下步骤去完成热塑膜的制作：

Next, we can use the following steps to complete the thermoplastic mask:

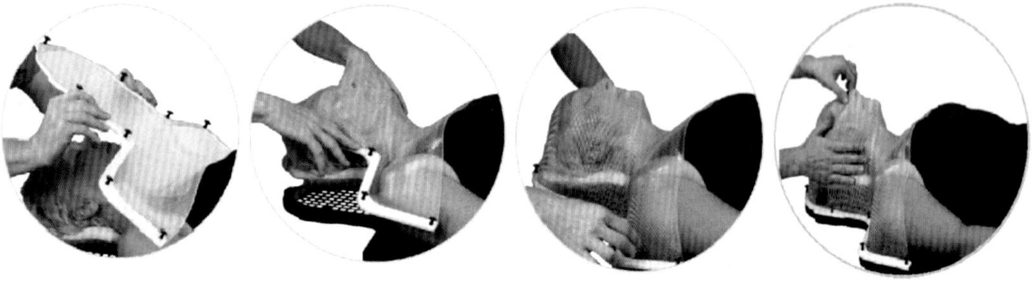

（1）取出我们专用的头颈部热塑膜置于水温为70 ℃的水箱中，加热时间以1 min为宜，时间过长或过短都会对热塑膜的正常使用有较大的影响。

Put out our dedicated head and neck thermoplastic mask in the water tank when the water temperature is 70 ℃. The heating time is 1 min advisable. Too long or too short time for the normal use of thermoplastic mask have a great influence.

（2）取出已加热好的热塑膜，用毛巾轻触，除去多余的水分。

Remove the mask that has been heated and gently touch it with a towel to remove excess water.

（3）按照如图的方式，进行热塑膜的制作。在整个制作过程中要保证患者没有过度的移动。

Make the thermoplastic mask according to the figure. Be sure that in the whole process of making the patient is not over moving.

（4）待热塑膜塑型完成后，参考技术标准，冷却时间为8 min 45 s。正常情况下，一般让患者静坐10 min为宜。在冷却的过程中要严密观察患者的头部，叮嘱患者切勿移动头部，以免对精确地塑型造成大的影响。如果发现患者的移动幅度较大，或者热塑膜的塑型没有达到预期效果，应立即将面罩取下并置于水箱中，重复以上操作，进行患者再定位。

After the plasticity of thermoplastic mask was completed, according to technology standard, the cooling time was 8 min 45 s. Normally, it is advisable for patients to sit for 10 min. In the process of cooling, the patient's head should be closely monitored and the patient should not move the head to affect the accuracy of the plastic. If it is found that the patient's movements are larger or thermoplastic film shape did not achieve the desired effect, the mask will be immediately removed and put into the tank. Repeat the above operation until finished the immobilization.

5 患者信息记录

(Patient Information Record)

待热塑膜制作完成后，所有的头颈部固定膜具就完成了。最后务必记录患者的详细信息于固定膜具上，包括患者使用过的Lok-Bar位置参数、头枕的类型、热塑膜的类型。

After the preparation of the thermoplastic mask, all the head-and-neck fixing mask were completed. Finally, it is important to record the patient's detailed information on the fixed mask, including the lok-bar position parameter patient's used, the type of pillow and the type of thermoplastic mask.

第4节　头颈部肿瘤碳离子放射治疗摆位标准操作流程
Standard Operating Procedure for Carbon Ion Radiotherapy Positioning of Head and Neck Tumor

作者：李文祺　陈东基　祁英　孟万斌　马霄云

1　根据患者信息，找出患者的面罩、颚部模具、头部框架、头枕

(According to the patient information, look for the patient's mask, jaw mold, head frame，pillow)

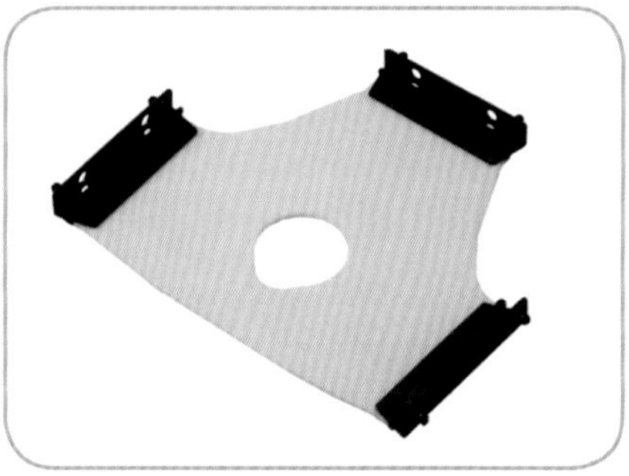

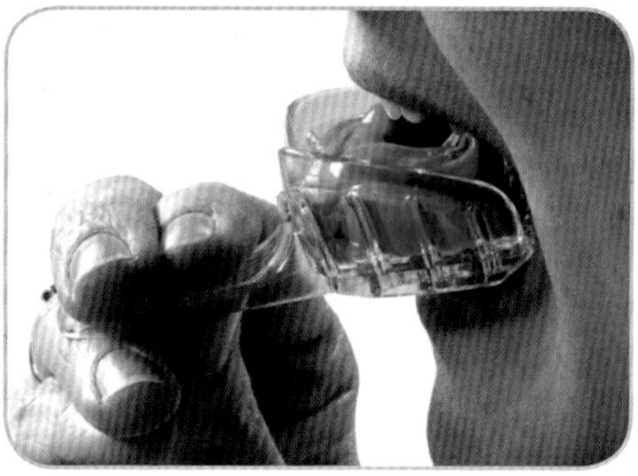

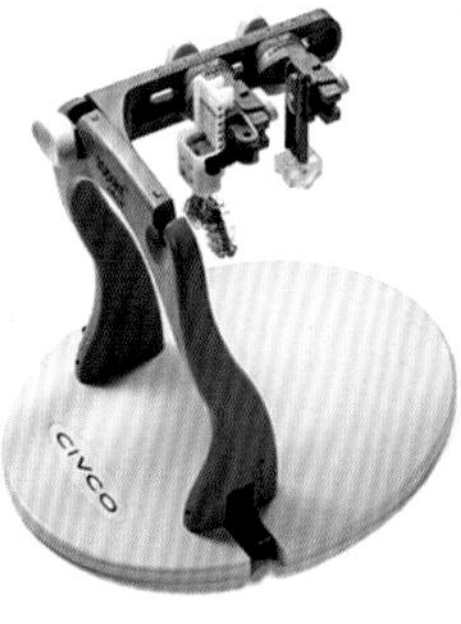

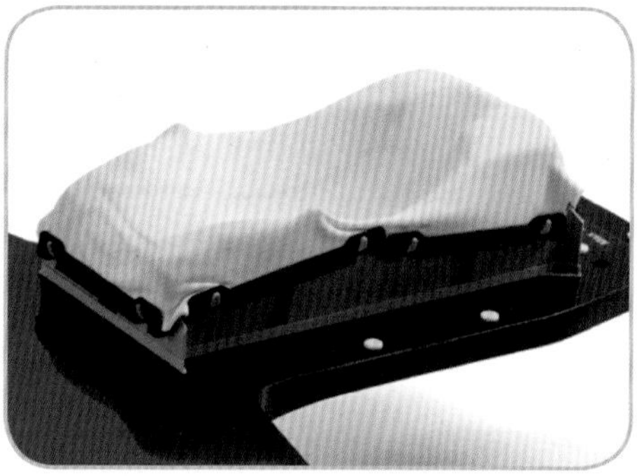

2　呼叫患者进入准备间

(Call the patient into the preparation room)

3　技师核对患者信息

(The technician checks the patient information)

4 患者更换衣服

(The patient changes clothes)

5 指挥患者躺到床上

(Command the patient lying on the bed)

6 根据体表标记将膜固定

(According to the body surface tag to fix film)

7 含入颚部模具

(The patient bite the jaw mold)

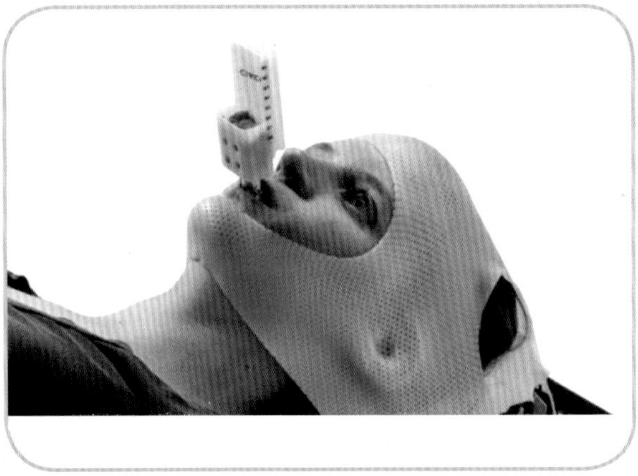

8 放置头部框架

(Put the head frame)

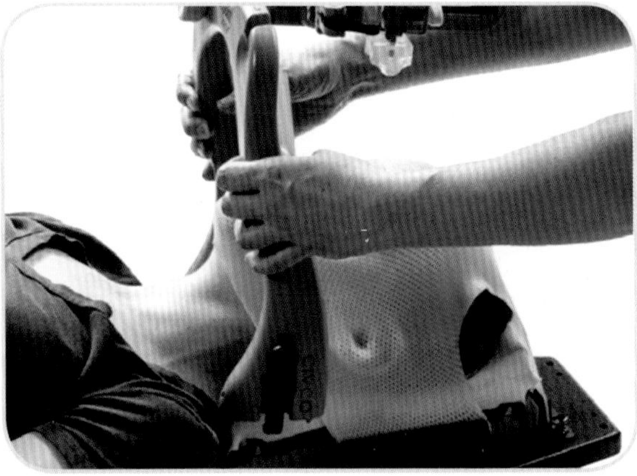

9 固定完毕
(Finished)

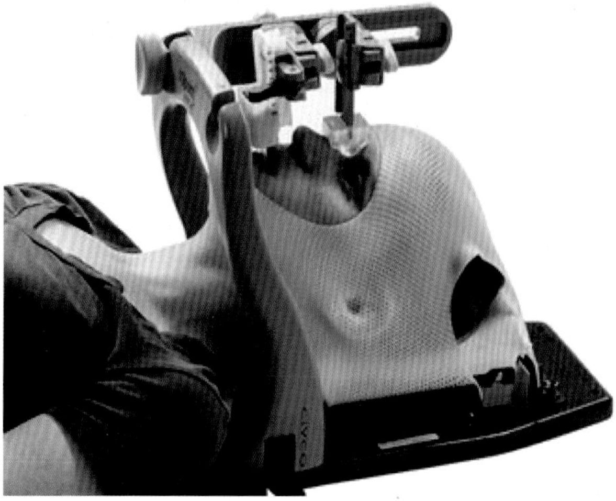

10 转运患者完成后，将患者和DR设备共同移动至治疗中心处
(After the delivery of the patient, the patient and the DR device are all moved to the center of the treatment.)

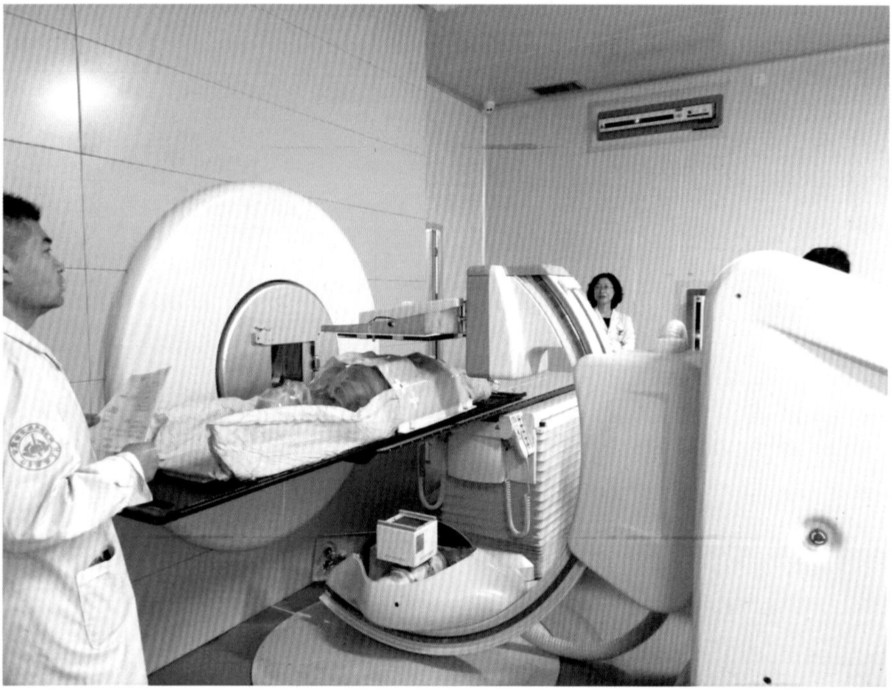

11 打开DR软件，输入相关参数

(Open the DR software and import the parameters)

距离1.8米时,柯尼卡板,东芝球管,CPI			距离1.2米时,柯尼卡板,东芝球管,CPI		
头颅(正)	80	20	头颅(正)	75	20
头颅(侧)	80	20	头颅(侧)	75	20

12 按曝光按钮（长按大约2～3 s）进行曝光拍片。拍摄完成后，将已经拍摄好的DR图像按患者姓名传送至ciGPS

[Press the exposure button (long press about 2–3 s) for exposure. After the shooting, the captured DR image should be sent to the ciGPS according to the patient's name.]

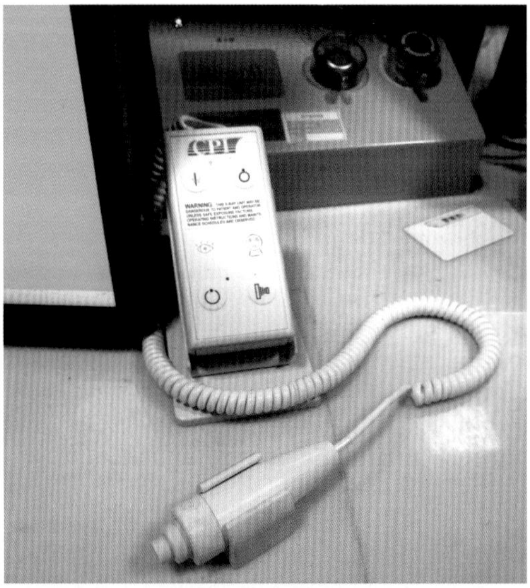

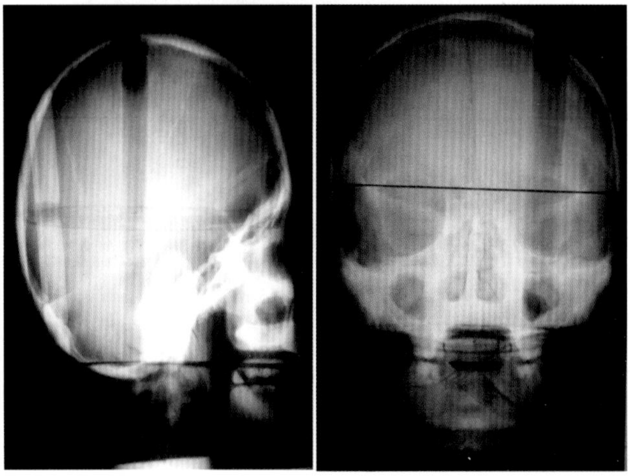

13　登录 ciGPS，导入患者数据，进行图像配准

（Sign into ciGPS, import patient data, and make image registration.）

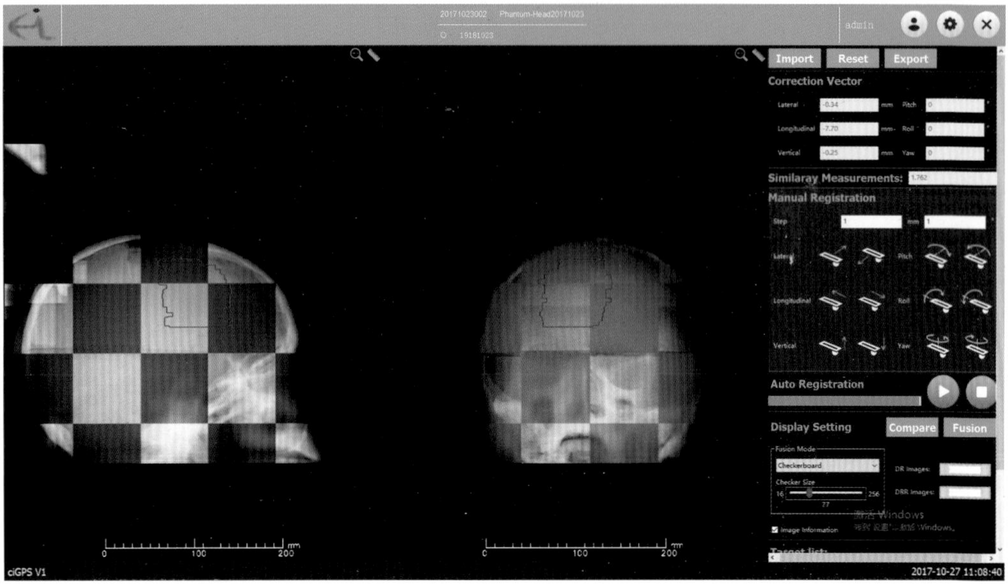

13.1　手动配准（Manual registration）

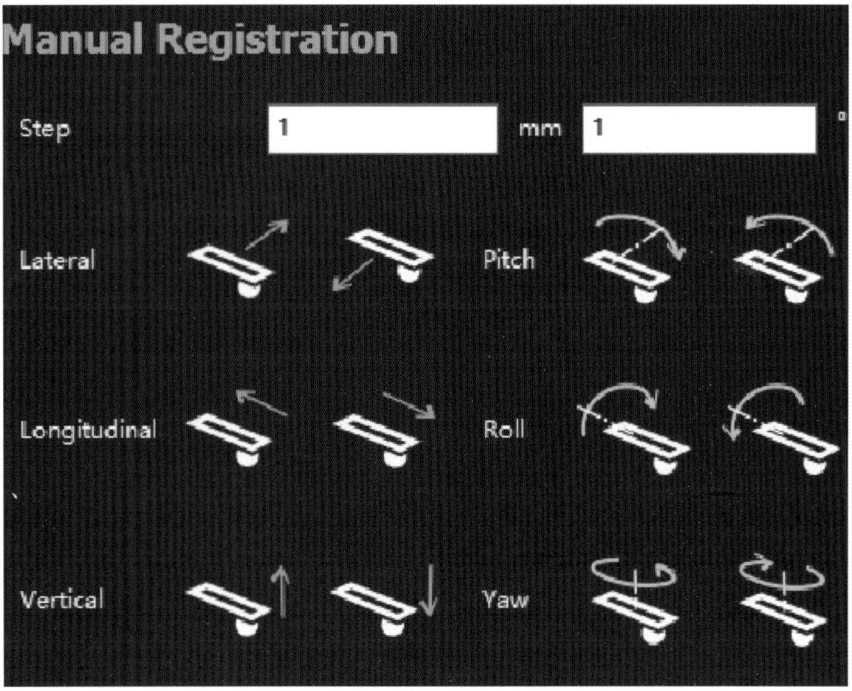

按下相应图标即可实现调整，step栏可设置每一次微调的幅度。

Press the corresponding icon to achieve the adjustment, step bar can be set to adjust the size of each time.

13.2 自动配准（Auto Registration）

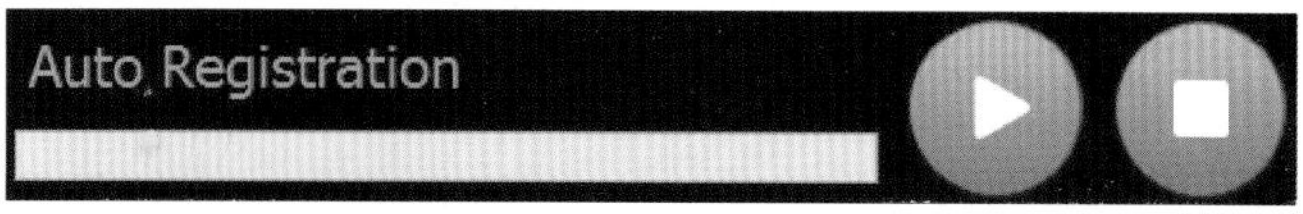

在Auto Registration栏点击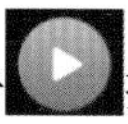按钮，开始配准。

Click the 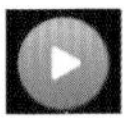 button in the Auto Registration column to start the registration.

14 配准移床完成后，进行再拍片验证，看是否配准正确。如有配准错误出现，可以重新进行配准，直至正确。

(After the registration bed is completed, verify the film to see if the registration is correct. If registration errors occur, you can do it again, until it's correct.)

第5节　胸部肿瘤患者碳离子放射治疗体位固定标准操作流程

Standard Operation Procedure for the Carbon Ion Radiotherapy Immobilization of Chest Tumor Patients

作者：李文祺　陈东基　祁英　孟万斌　马霄云

1　将转运托架、真空袋平展放在床上，并用lock-bar固定，用卡扣将床板和转运托架固定。

(Place the transfer board and vacuum bag on the bed, and use lock-bar to fix it.Fix the bed on the transfer board by catch.)

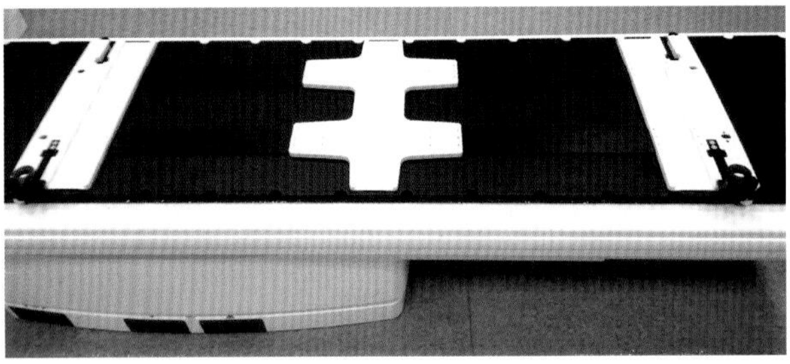

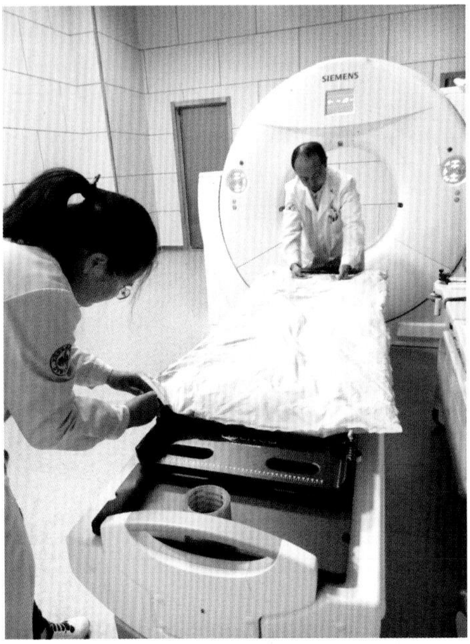

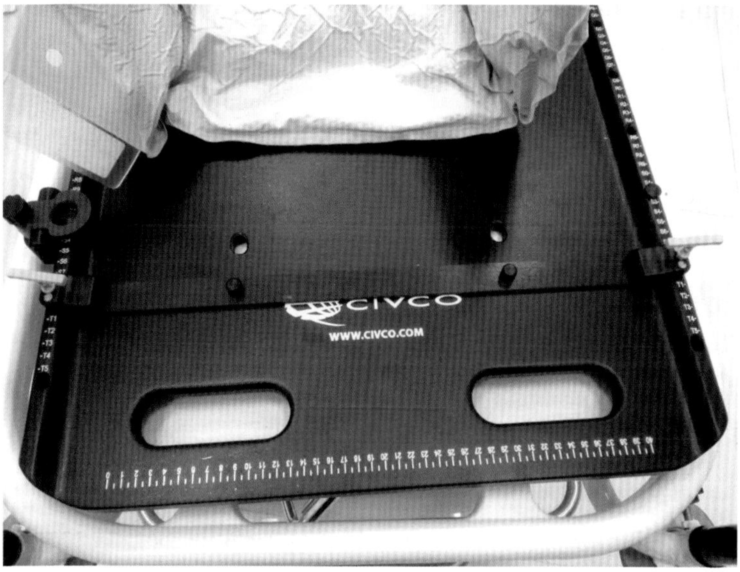
CIVCO
WWW.CIVCO.COM

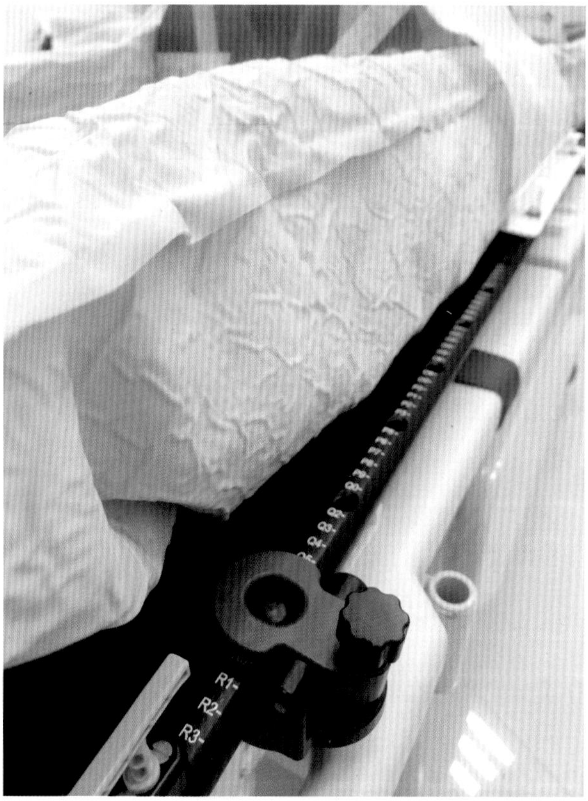
R1-
R2-
R3-

2 两名技师核对病人信息，确认无误，令病人躺在真空袋上。
(Two technicians check the patient information, if it is confirmed to be correct, order the patient to lie on the vacuum bag.)

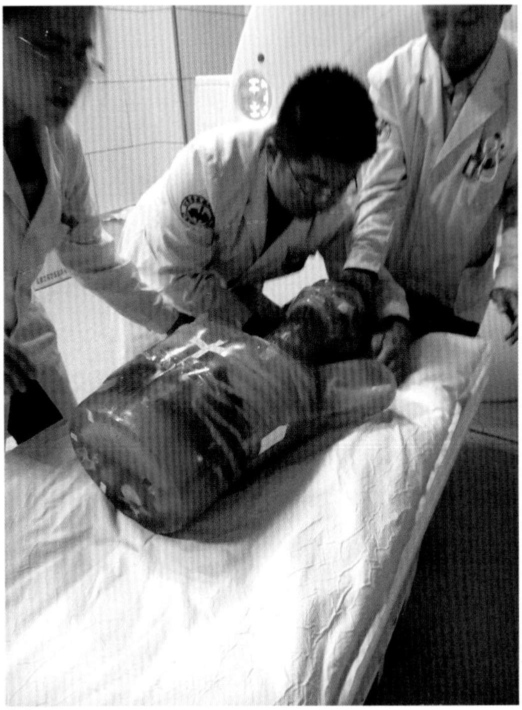

3 一名技师将热塑膜放进70 ℃恒温水箱中软化。
(One technician puts the plastic film into the 70 ℃ constant temperature water tank to make it soft.)

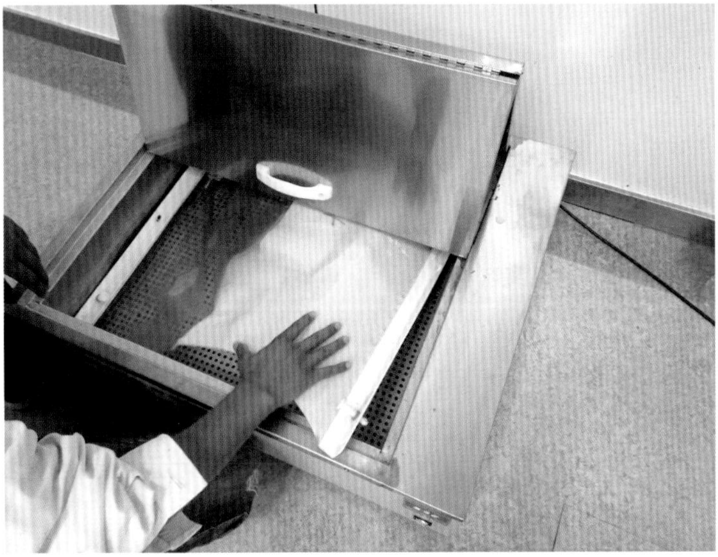

4 另一名技师告知病人注意事项，嘱咐其在体膜制作期间不可活动
(Another technician tells the patient to be inactive during this period.)

5 在病人身下放置头枕。
(Place the pillow under the patient.)

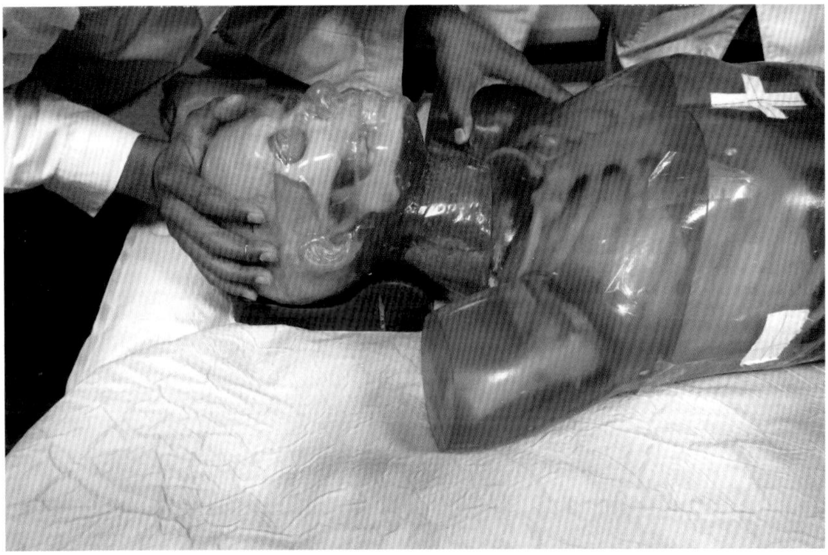

6 两名技师用手按压真空袋，令之贴合患者的身体。
(Two technicians press the vacuum bag to make it fit the patient's body.)

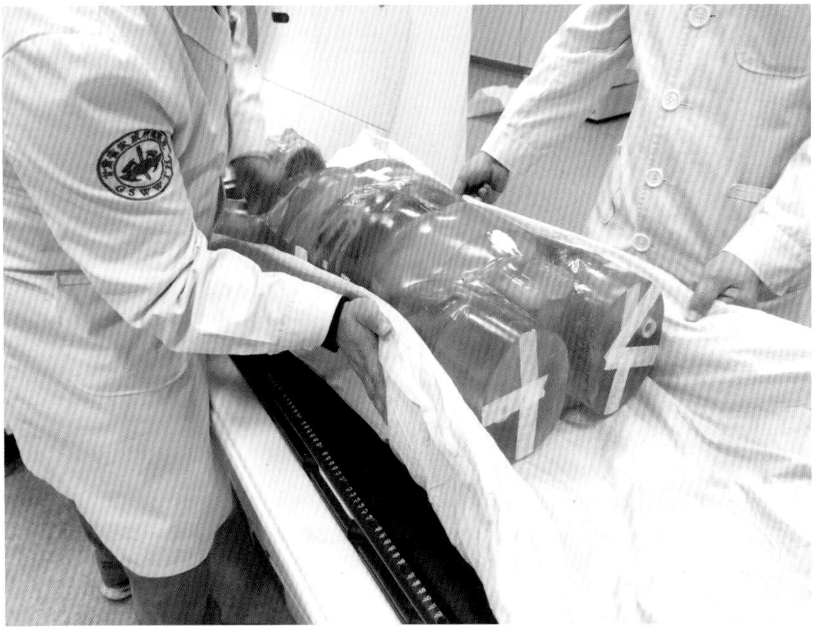

7 用真空泵对真空袋抽气，至负大气压0.08 MPa。

(Technician uses the pump to evacuate the vacuum bag until the negative pressure is 0.08 MPa.)

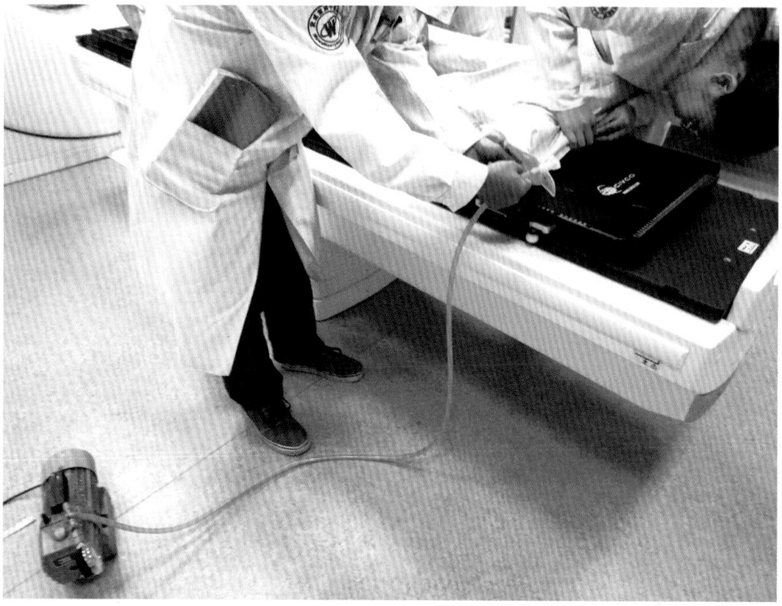

8 取出软化的热塑膜，放置于病人身体中央，两名技师同时在两侧拉扯。

(Pick up the softened thermoplastic film, placed it on the patient's body center, two technicians standing on both sides, pulling at the same time.)

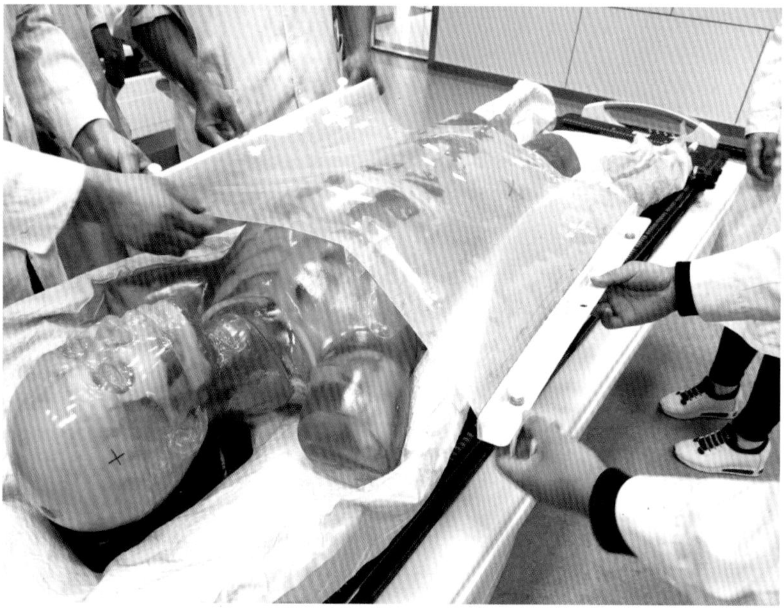

9 选取床板两侧相同编号孔洞，将插销插入，固定。

(Select the same number of holes on both sides of the bed board, insert the pin, fix.)

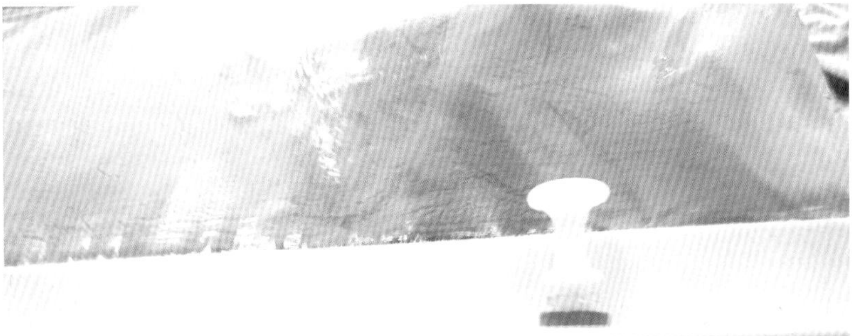

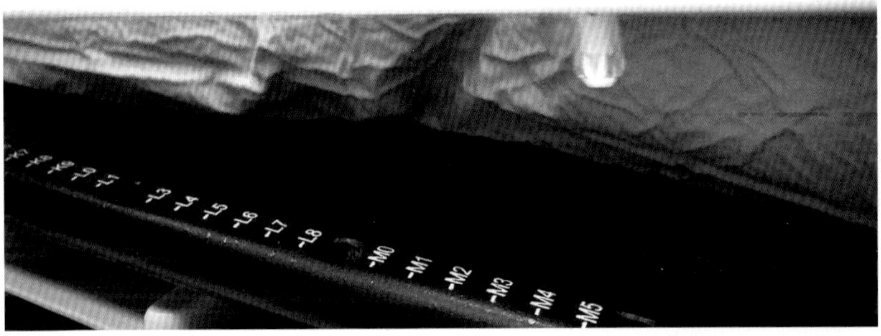

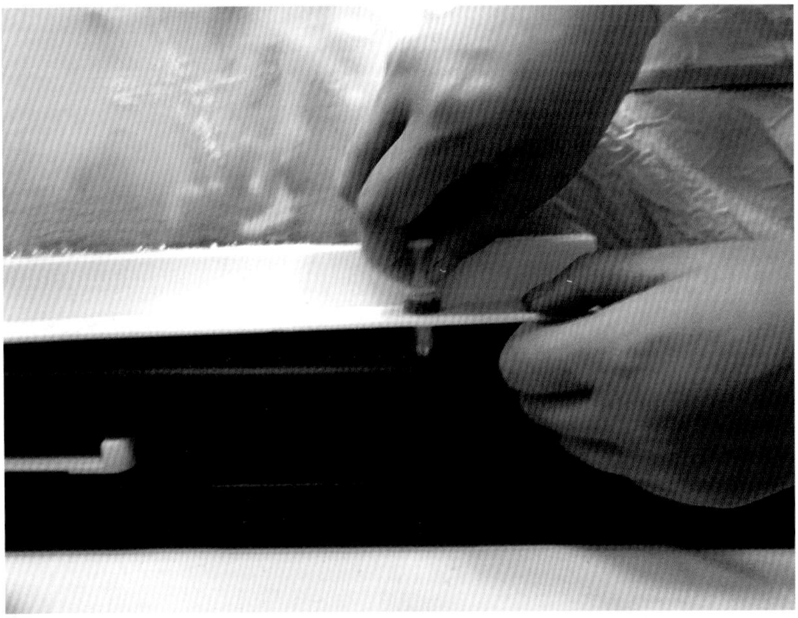

10 推动转运车到CT床旁边，并与CT床平行

(Push the transporter to the CT bed which is to be parallel to the CT bed.)

11 在CT床上插入转运板

(Insert the transfer plate on CT bed)

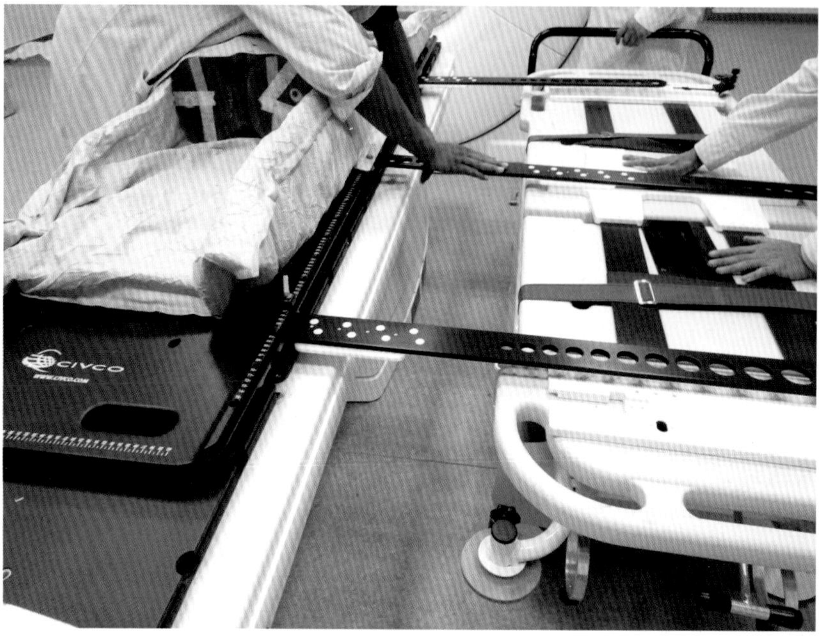

12 调整CT床和转运床到同一高度

(Adjust the CT bed and transporter to the same height.)

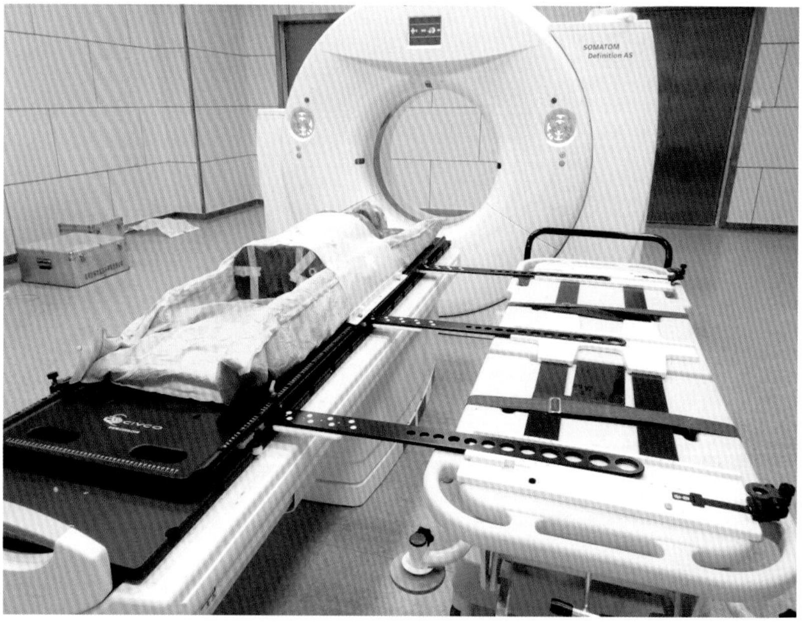

13 松开卡扣，将病人和真空袋一起推到转运车上

（Unlock the fixed catch, push the patient and vacuum bag to the transporter.）

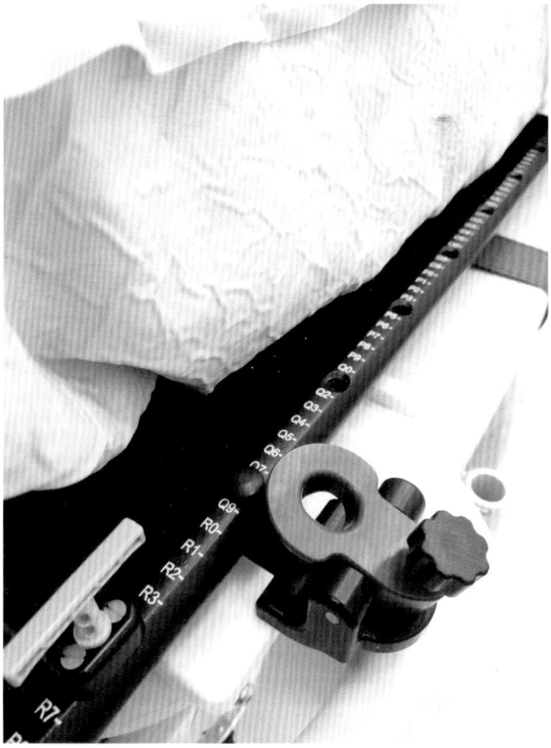

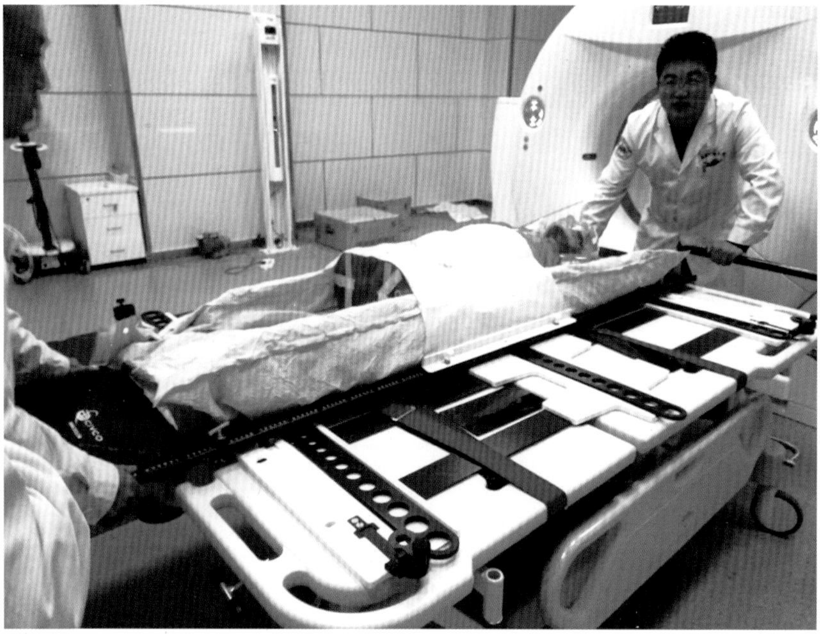

14　取下转运板，推动转运车到准备间

（Remove the transfer plate and push the transporter to the preparation room.）

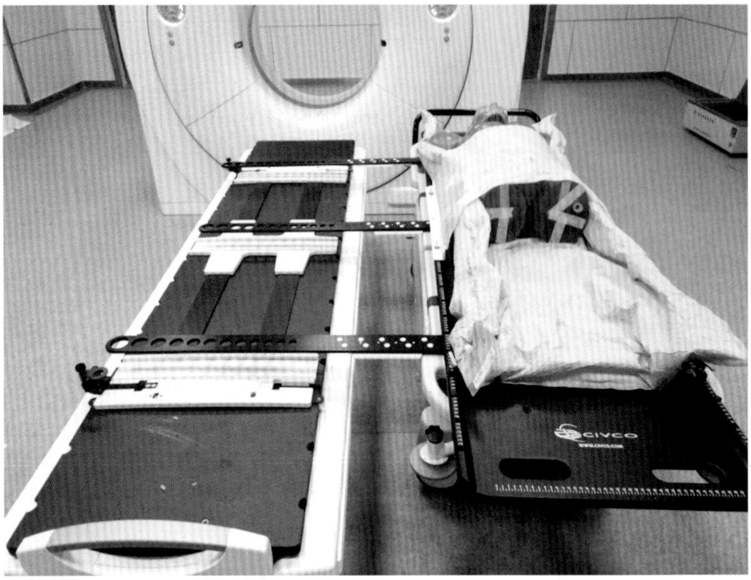

15　等待热塑膜冷却硬化后，取下。

（Wait for the thermoplastic film to cool and then remove it.）

16　协助护士搀扶病人下床。

（Help patients get out of bed with the nurse.）

第6节　胸、腹部肿瘤碳离子放射治疗摆位标准操作流程
Standard Operation Procedure for Carbon Ion Radiotherapy Positioning of Chest and Abdomen Tumor

作者：鲁会祥　祁英　孟万斌　马霄云

胸部肿瘤主要有胸壁肿瘤、纵隔肿瘤和肺部肿瘤。腹部肿瘤主要有腹壁肿瘤、胃癌、大肠癌等。患者摆位中一般采用头先进仰卧位、头先进俯卧位、头先进左侧卧位或者头先进右侧卧位。

Chest tumors are mainly chest wall tumors, mediastinal tumors and lung tumors. Abdominal tumors mainly include abdominal wall tumor, gastric cancer, large intestine cancer and so on. Patient positioning is generally head first supine position, head first prone position, head first left lateral position or head first right lateral position.

从便于重复治疗的目标出发，使患者治疗面从正面接近0°或90°的束流方向，容易接近治疗机架准直器。治疗摆位由两名放疗技师操作，具体摆位流程如下：

For the goal of repeated treatment, the patient treatment surface is easily accessible from the treatment frame collimator in the beam direction from the front close to 0° or 90°. Treatment positioning is done by two radiotherapy technicians, the specific process is as follows:

1　病人在更衣间在医生的指导下更换一次性无纺布无菌衣，如下图所示。对于胸腹部肿瘤患者，建议上身裸露，仅更换下身裤子。

(Patients replace disposable non - woven sterile clothing in the locker room, as shown below. For patients with chest and abdomen tumors, upper body is suggested to be nudity, only replace the lower body pants.)

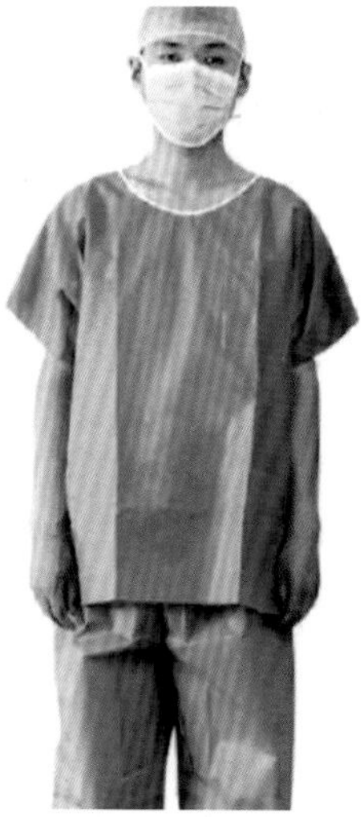

2　根据患者姓名、基本信息、临床诊断的腹部肿瘤位置，核对、使用摆位板、负压袋和热塑膜等其他辅助用具。

(According to the basic information and the

patient's name, the clinical diagnosis of abdomen tumor location, check and use positioning board, vacuum bag and other auxiliary equipment such as thermoplastic film.)

3 两名放疗技师在治疗床左右两侧，利用激光线对好体位固定板刻度线、负压袋和患者肢体上的标记线，并适当微调。

(Two radiotherapy technicians sit on the left and right sides of the treatment bed, make use of laser line on the good fixed - line calibration marks, negative pressure bags and the patient's body mark line, and fine-tuning.)

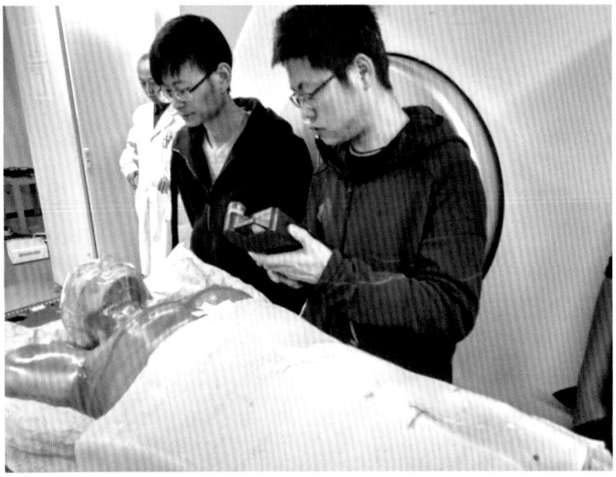

4 将热塑膜根据标记位置固定在患者治疗部位，再次利用激光线使左侧、右侧和中间的治疗靶线对齐。

(According to the marking position to fix thermoplastic film at the patient's treatment site, use the laser line to align the treatment target lines on the left, right and middle again.)

5 DR位置确认

(Location confirmation)

DR设备为患者位置确认的主要硬件设备。如图，在患者的转运完成后，我们按照患者的摆位要求，将患者置于需治疗的等中心点处（图①），按患者治疗所需的要求，将DR设备操作控制至等中心点处（图②③④）。按照位置确认的要求，我们采取正交验证，即水平和垂直两个正交方向（图③④）。在控制DR设备的过程中，要密切注视DR臂与治疗床之间是否有碰床现象。

The DR device is the main hardware device for patient location confirmation. As shown in the figure, after the completion of the patient's transport, we set the patient in accordance with the position requirements of the patient. The patient is placed at the treatment center (Figure

①). According to the requirements of patient treatment, the DR equipment operation is controled to the isocenter (Figure ② ③ ④). In accordance with the requirements of location confirmation, we take orthogonal verification, that is, horizontal and vertical orthogonal direction (Figure ③ ④). In the process of controlling the DR device, it is necessary to strictly observe whether there is a collision between the DR arm and the treatment bed.

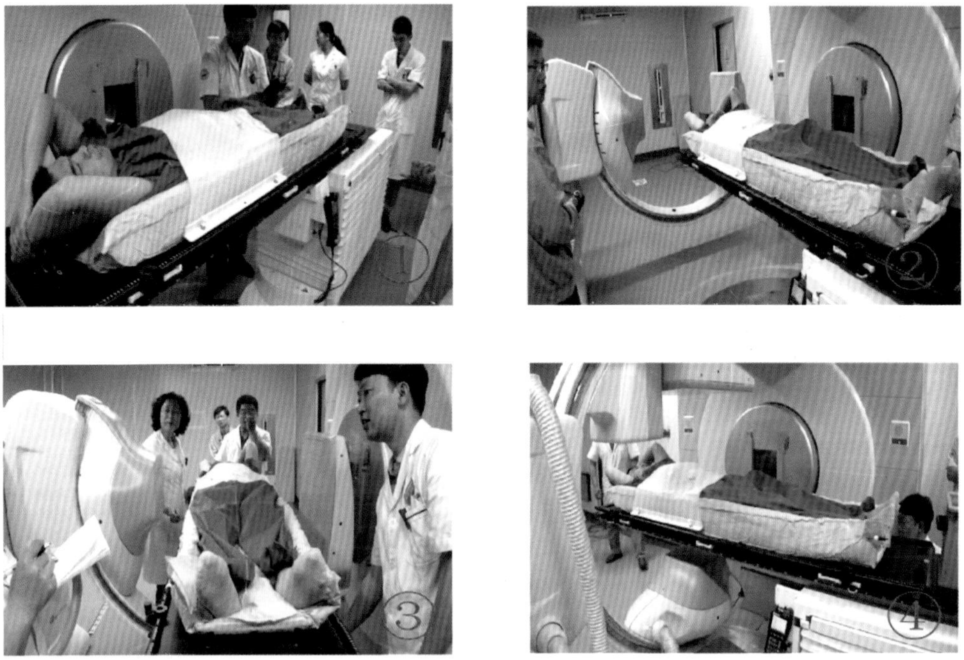

6 DR 曝光

(DR exposure)

曝光拍摄完成后，将已经拍摄好的DR图像按患者姓名传送至ciGPS。

After the shooting of the exposure is completed, sent the DR image to ciGPS by patient's name.

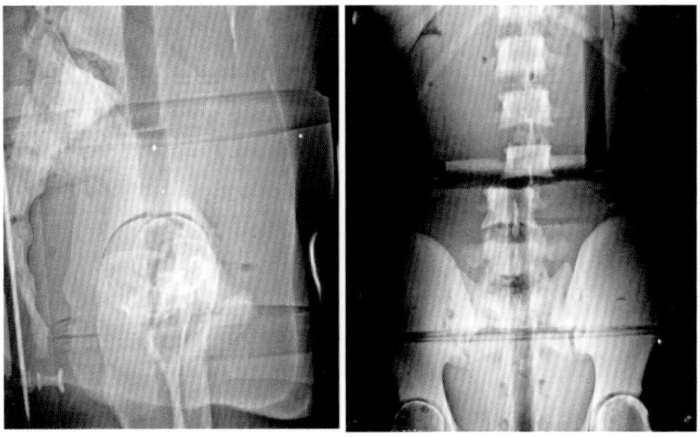

7 运行

(ciGPS Run ciGPS)

重离子摆位验证系统通过治疗前定位DR系统产生的患者DR影像与治疗计划CT数据生成的数字影像重建图像（DRR）的配准，计算治疗床的偏移量来引导患者摆位过程，确保治疗位置的准确性。导入患者数据，数据包含CT图像、RTSS、RTPlan、两张DR图像和两张DRR图像。

The carbon ion placement verification system registers the positioning DR data of the patient and the CT data of the treatment plan generated by the pre-treatment positioning DR system and calculates the displacement of the treatment table to guide the patient to position and ensure the accuracy of the treatment position. Import patient data, the data including CT images, RTSS, RTPlan, two DR images and two DRR images.

8 重置DRR图像至初始状态有手动配准和自动配准两种配准方式，配准结束后可以导出到ois系统。

(There are manual registration and automatic registration to reset the DRR image to the initial state. After the registration, the DRR image can be exported to the ois system.)

8.1 患者信息导入（Patient information import）

如下图是对患者进行管理的主要功能按钮，ciGPS包含导入数据（Import）、导出数据（Export）和重置参数（Reset）3个功能。

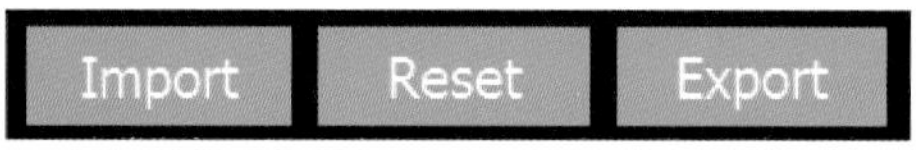

Import：用来导入患者数据

Reset：用来重置配准操作

Export：用来导出治疗床移动参数到OIS系统

导入数据的操作步骤如下：

（1）点击Import打开导入界面

（2）点击Browse打开文件管理器

（3）选择要导入的数据所在文件夹

（4）点击select folder按钮，数据路径显示在FileName内

（5）点击Import按钮即可导入

The following figure shows the main function buttons for patient management. ciGPS includes three functions: Import, Export and Reset.

The steps for importing data are as follows:

（1）Click Import to open the import interface

（2）Click Browse to open the file manager

（3）Select the folder where the data you want to import

（4）Click the select folder button, the data path is displayed in the FileName

（5）Click the Import button to import

8.2　图像配准（Image registration）

ciGPS提供了自动配准和手动配准两种方法。

ciGPS provides both automatic registration and manual registration methods.

（1）手动配准（Manual Registration）

Manual Registration是设置手动配准参数以及进行配准操作的控制面板。手动配准参数包括每次平移的距离和每次旋转的角度。

Manual Registration is to set the manual registration parameters and the registration operation of the control panel. Manual registration parameters include the distance of each translation and the angle of each rotation.

（2）自动配准（Automatic Registration）

Auto Registration是自动配准区域，包含配准进度条、开始配准按钮和终止配准按钮，如图所示。

Auto Registration is an auto registration area that contains the registration progress bar, the start registration button and the end registration button, as shown in the figure.

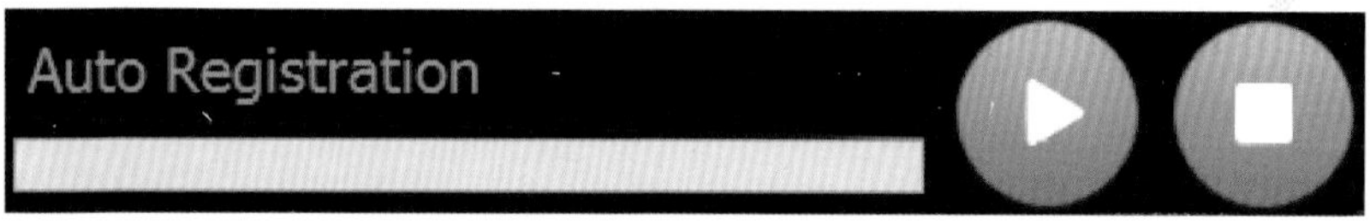

开启自动配准：

（1）点击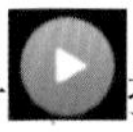按钮，开始配准

（2）DRR图像位置开始变动，偏移量和配准误差的值变化

（3）配准完成，提示【Auto Registration completed!】

在配准的过程中，如出现故障如需重新摆位等情况，也可以终止自动配准：

（4）点击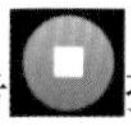按钮，

（5）点击OK，停止配准/点击Cancel，继续自动配准

Turn on automatic registration:

（1）Click the 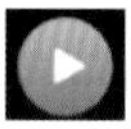 button to start registration

（2）DRR image position begins to change, the offset and registration error value changes

（3）The registration is completed, prompted 【Auto Registration completed! 】

In the registration process, such as the need for re - positioning because of accident, etc., you can also terminate the automatic registration:

（4）Click the 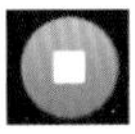 button,

（5）Click OK, stop registration / click Cancel, continue automatic registration

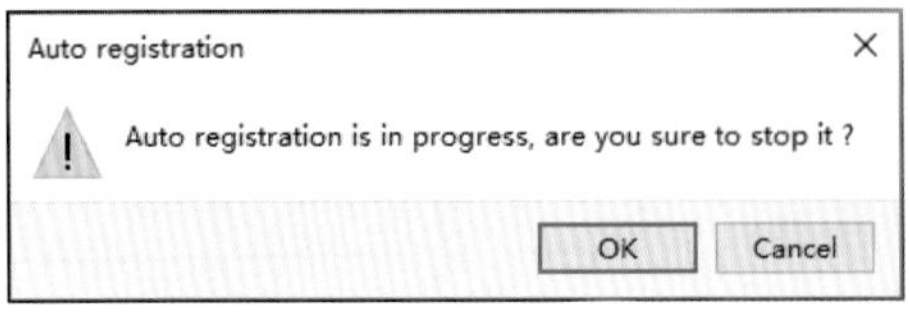

9 配准完成

(Registration completed)

如果是手动配准，确保配准正确，主管医生已经确认签字后，方可执行治疗。

If use manual registration, ensure that the registration is correct, treatment can be carried out only after the competent doctor has confirmed and signature.

10 再次告知患者在治疗期间的相关注意事项，摆位技师关闭防护门，准备实施治疗。

(Inform the patient during the treatment again. The technician closes the protective door, be ready to implement the treatment.)

第7节　腹部、盆腔肿瘤碳离子放射治疗体位固定标准操作流程

Standard Operation Procedure for Carbon Ion Radiotherapy Treatment Immobilization of Abdomen and Chest Tumor Patient

作者：鲁会祥　祁英　孟万斌　马霄云

腹部肿瘤患者的体位固定相对于头颈部和胸部的略微简单，与传统光子放疗采用相同的固定模式及技术。但是考虑到碳离子放射治疗较为精准，故我们采用全身型真空负压袋以及无网孔热塑膜以起到对全身固定的作用，提高碳离子放射治疗精确度。下面就腹部患者体位固定的技术要求做详细的介绍。

The immobilization of the abdominal tumor patients is slightly simpler than that of the head and neck and the chest tumor patients, and the same fixed pattern and technique are used as the traditional photon radiotherapy. But considering the accuracy of carbon ion radiotherapy, we use a systemic vacuum bag and a non - mesh thermoplastic film. In order to improve the accuracy of carbon ion treatment, it can be fixed to the whole body. The following is a detailed introduction to the technical requirements of the immobilization of the abdominal tumor patients.

由于盆腔肿瘤患者治疗部位在身体中下段，患者体位固定中一般采用头先进仰卧位、头先进俯卧位、头先进左侧卧位或者头先进右侧卧位。选择束流穿射正常组织距离最短的体位，不仅有利于提高放疗的精确性，更有利于减少盆腔、下腹部肠道、双肾、膀胱、股骨头等器官的受照剂量，降低正常组织的副反应。

As the pelvic cancer patients treatment part is in the lower segment of body, the patient immobilization is generally the first head supine position, the first prone position, the first left lateral position or the first right lateral position. Select the beam through the normal body tissue distance shortest position not only help to improve the accuracy of radiotherapy, but also help to reduce the dose of pelvic, lower abdomen intestinal, kidney, bladder, femoral head and other organs, reduce side effects on the normal tissue.

腹部、盆腔肿瘤患者的体位固定大致可分为两步：

The immobilization of the abdominal tumor patients can be roughly divided into two steps.

（1）真空负压袋塑型（Vacuum vacuum bag plasticity）；

（2）热塑膜塑型（Thermoplastic film plasticity）。

1　真空负压袋

我院采用的真空负压袋由美国CIVCO公司提供的，按我院要求特殊定制的尺寸为80 cm×200 cm全身型真空负压袋。内部由小的聚苯乙烯珠填充，真空垫在病人周围形成一个坚硬的、舒适的襁褓，以起到保护病人和固定病人的作用。

The vacuum vacuum bag used by our hospital is provided by the CIVCO company of the United States. According to the special custom size of our hospital, the vacuum vacuum bag is 80 cm×200 cm body type. The inside is filled with small polystyrene beads, and the vacuum pad forms a hard and comfortable baby around the patient to play a role in protecting patients and fixing patients.

1.1　Lok-Bar

真空负压袋的制作，首先由固定负压袋的固定条Lok-Bar开始。这是专用于SBRT板上的一种锁定条，由碳纤维材料制成，该材料符合碳离子放射治疗的材料要求。

The making of vacuum bag is started from the fixed bar Lok-Bar. This is a locking strip designed for SBRT plate, made of carbon fiber material that meets the material requirements for carbon ion radio therapy.

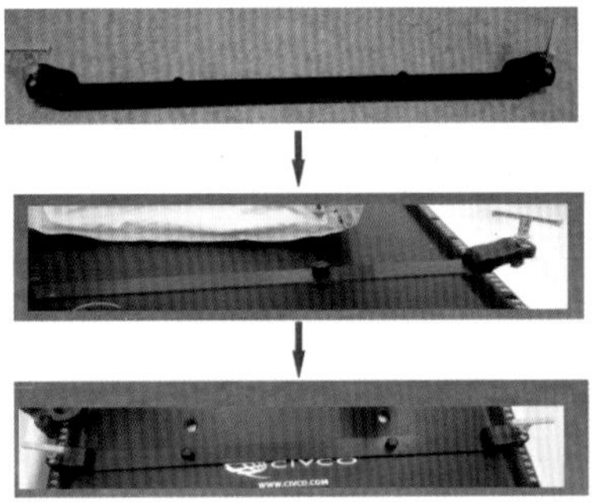

1.2　真空负压袋

1.2.1　锁定真空负压袋到Lok-Bar条（Lock the vacuum bag to the Lok-Bar）

因为Lok-Bar和真空负压袋也是配套使用的，所以Lok-Bar上的小凸球和真空负压袋上的小凹槽组成锁定卡扣。但是在通常情况下，因为真空负压袋在抽真空时会适量地缩短，导致原来的锁定卡扣滑脱，经反复实验和测试，最好的距离是在Lok-Bar的位置，向内（缩短）20 cm，这样一来，当真空负压袋抽真空缩短时，刚好达到预设的长度，锁定卡扣也不会滑脱。

Because the Lok-Bar and vacuum bag are also included, the small tabs on the Lok-Bar and the small grooves in the vacuum bag create a locking tab. However, under normal circumstances, the vacuum bag vacuum will be shortened when it is pumped, which will lead to the original lock snap off, so after repeated experiments and tests, the best distance is the location of the Lok - Bar to the inside (shortened) 20 cm, this way, when the vacuum bag vacuum shortening, just reach the preset length, the locking buckle will not slip.

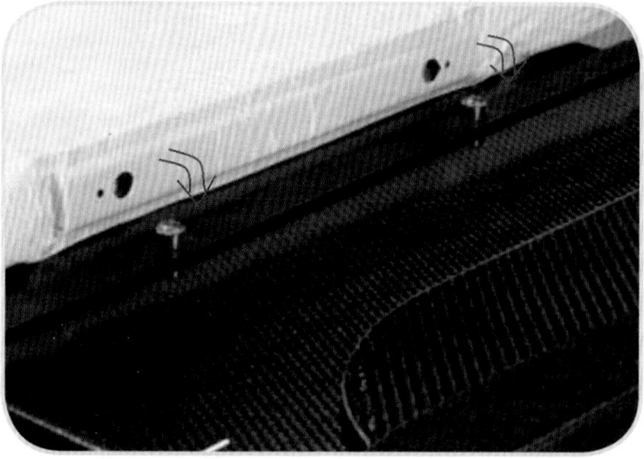

1.2.2 病人预定位（The patient pre-positioning）

真空负压袋准备就绪后，就要进行病人的预定位工作。让已经更换好病员服准备就绪的病人脱掉拖鞋，上床躺在真空负压袋上，调整病人的体位，取尽可能的水平仰卧位，双手置于头顶，以病人最舒适、保持时间最长的仰卧姿势为最佳。病人的预定位工作基本完成之后，按照患者的头部的位置以及头颅的大小，选择合适的头枕置于患者的颅底。

When vacuum vacuum bag is ready, it is necessary for the patient's pre-positioning work. So that patients who has wear the patient suits ready to take off the slippers, go to bed in a vacuum bag, adjust the patient's position, take the supine position as possible, his hands placed on the head. The supine position is best for the patients which is the most comfort, and can deep the longest time. When the patient's pre - positioning work is basically completed, according to the patient's head position, and the size of the skull, select the appropriate pillow placed in the patient's skull base.

1.2.3 真空负压袋（Vacuum bag）

真空负压袋的制作和传统光子放疗真空负压袋的制作技术要求相同，我们可根据光子放疗的经验去完成真空负压袋的制作。具体的步骤可总结如下：

Vacuum vacuum bag's making is the same to the traditional photon radiotherapy vacuum bag manufacturing technology require, so we can complete the vacuum bag according to photon radiotherapy experience. The specific steps can be summarized as follows:

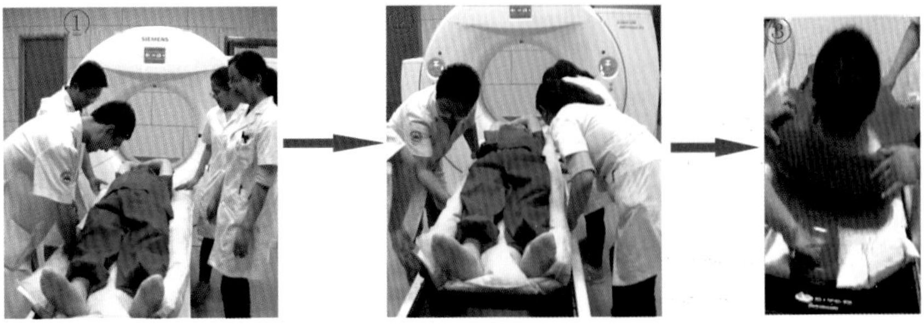

（1）在患者于负压袋最正中的情况下，卷起负压袋的边缘部分，紧贴于患者两侧，因为全身型负压袋比光子使用的负压袋长很多，所以目前的人员配置为4人协同完成。

When the patient is in the most positive position of the vacuum bag, roll up the edge of the vacuum bag and put it on both sides of the patient. The whole body vacuum bag is much longer than the ordinary vacuum bag, so it need the 4 people to collaboratively complete.

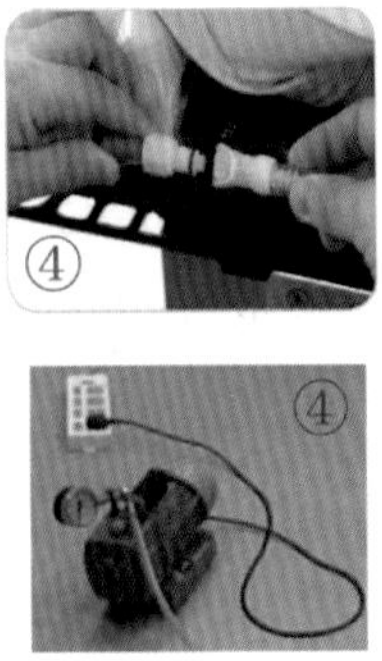

十分钟后

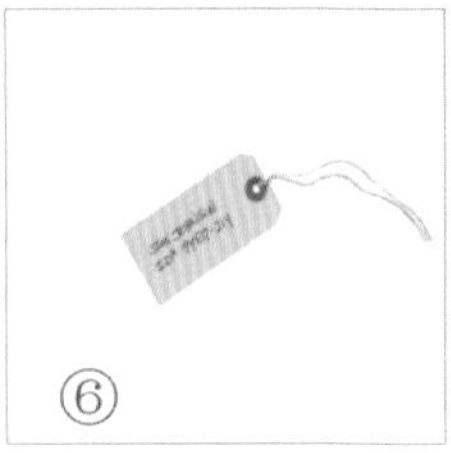

患者信息记录单

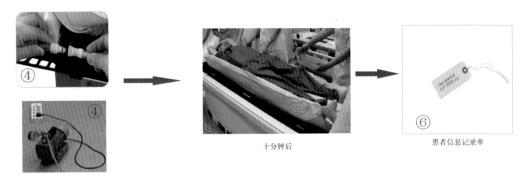

（2）真空负压袋初步塑型后，打开气泵，连接阀门，进行抽真空。这个阶段是最为关键的阶段，操作人员要仔细观察真空袋的硬化过程，确保真空袋每个部位的硬化都是我们预设的形状。

After the vacuum bag primary shapes, open the air pump, connect the valve, vacuum. This stage is the most critical stage, the operator should carefully observe the hardening process of the vacuum bag to ensure that each part of the vacuum bag is hardened to our default shape.

（3）确保真空袋的制作满足临床需求，完成后关闭气泵。

Make sure that the vacuum bag is made to meet clinical requirements and shut down the pump after it is done.

（4）制作完成后记录该真空负压袋的信息。真空负压袋有自己配套使用的便捷标签，我们应该详细记录患者的信息、真空袋气压、患者头枕型号、Lok-Bar index。

After the completion of the making, record the vacuum bag information. There is a convenient label for the vacuum bag. We should record patient information, vacuum bag pressure, patient pillow model, Lok-Bar index.

2 固定模具
(Fix mold)

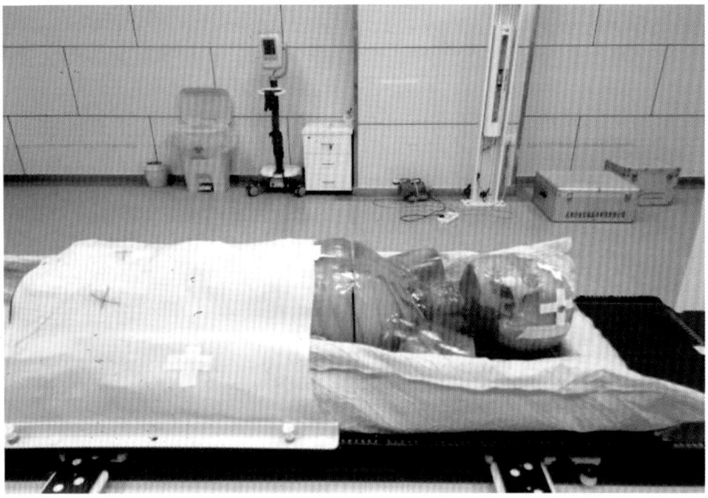

操作流程如下：

Operation procedure is as follows:

（1）将准备好的腹膜放入恒温水箱（75 ℃）中加热，使其由硬变软可以随意拉伸。

Put the prepared peritoneum into a constant temperature water tank （75 degrees Celsius）to heat it, so that it can be soft from the hard to stretch.

（2）将烫好的腹膜根据病人腹部病灶的位置趁热固定在病人身上（如上图所示）

According to the location of the patient' s pelvic lesions, fix peritoneum on the patient' s body (as shown in the figure).

（3）过十到十五分钟等到体膜收缩变凉，无自然形变时将模具取下，操作完毕。

After ten to fifteen minutes, if the body membrane contraction cool and no natural deformation, remove it. The operation is finished.

第8节　碳离子放射治疗CT定位标准操作流程
Standard Operating Procedure for CT Localization in Carbon Ion Radiotherapy

作者：杨晓东　祁英　孟万斌　马霄云

CT是目前临床依赖的重要检查手段之一，造影剂注射能对多个病种进行检查。放疗从二维发展到三维，治疗精度大大提升，其中CT也起到重大作用。我们现在用的CT的型号为SOMATOM DEFINITION AS 64。以下为CT在放疗中的具体作用和流程。

CT is one of the important methods of clinical dependence at present. Injection of contrast agent can be used to check multiple diseases. Radiotherapy has been developed from 2D-CRT to 3D-CRT and the treatment accuracy has been greatly improved. CT also plays a significant role. The CT model type we use now is SOMATOM DEFINITION AS 64. The following is to explain the specific function and use procedure of CT in radiotherapy.

1　启动系统
(Starting up system)

1.1　开机（Starting up）

CT机的总电源一般都处于连接状态，开机时，直接按下手操作板上的¤（power）键，机器进入开机画面。（power键上方的是计算机开机键，单独按下此键时只开启计算机，机架不会启动，最上面的键是强制启动键，机器出现故障、启动失败时可按下此键。）另外，操作面板上还集成了麦克风和听筒，可根据情况跟患者交流。

The total power supply of the CT is generally connected. When need starting up, press the power button directly on the operating panel. The machine enters the boot screen.(On the top of the power button is the computer boot key, which only turn on the computer when the key is pressed. The gantry will not move, and the top key is the forced start button, which can be pressed when there is an accident or the machine fails to start.) In addition, the operating panel also integrates the microphone and the receiver, which can communicate with the patient according to the situation.

1.2 启动检查系统（Start checking system）

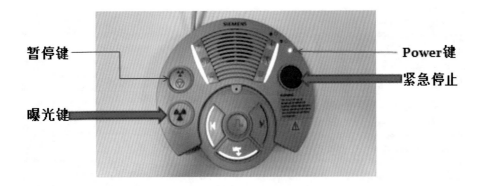

暂停键：Stop button

曝光键：Exposure button

紧急停止：Emergency stop

待机器进入检查界面，此时会自动弹出Checkup对话框，点击Checkup后按下Start键进行预热。注意：CT闲置4小时要做一次calibration.

After the boot screen, the machine will be a check interface, the dialog box of checkups will automatically pop up, after click it, press the Start button to preheat.

tip: CT is idle for 4 hours for a calibration.

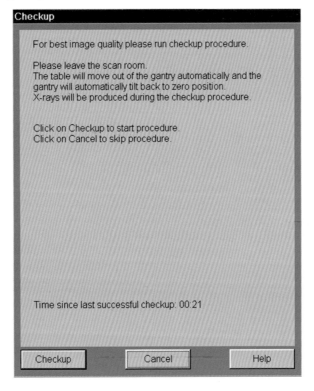

2 准备病人

(Prepare the patient)

2.1 对病人进行登记（Register the patient）

（1）点击此图标出现相应登记病人的对话框。

Click this icon to lead to the patient's dialog box.

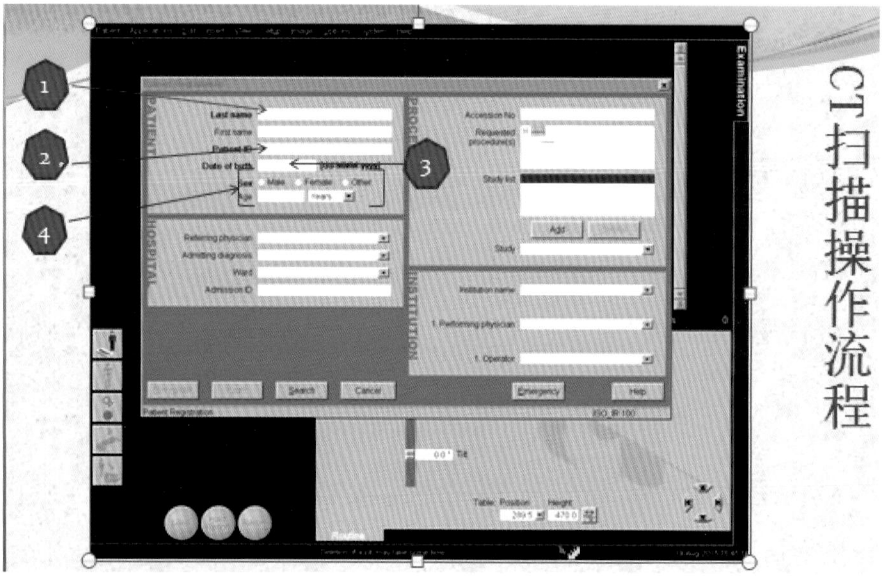

（2）填写所有强制输入项（姓名、ID、出生日期、性别和年龄）。

Fill in all mandatory entries (name, ID, date of birth, gender and age).

（3）点击确认检查。

Click confirmation to check.

2.2 选择扫描方案（Select the scanning scheme）

（1）在病人模式对话框中，选择所要进行扫描的部位（例如：头部、胸部、腹部、盆部 等）。

Select the site to be scanned in the patient mode dialog box (e.g. head, chest, abdomen, pelvis, etc.).

（2）在选择列表中选择所需的扫描方案。

Select the desired scan option in the selection list.

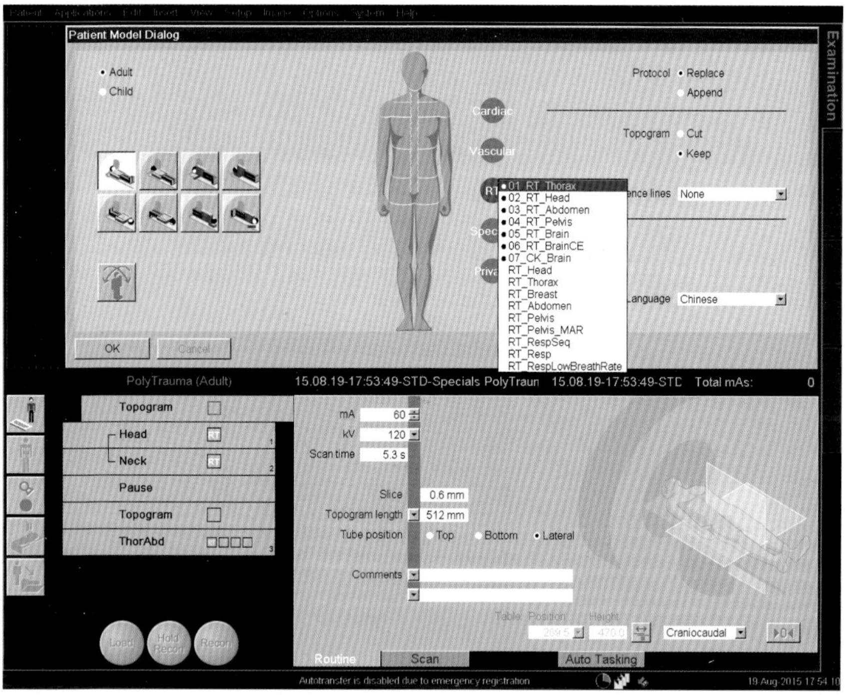

（3）点击确认。

Click on the confirmation.

2.3 病人定位（The patient's positioning）

（1）在机架操作界面上，保持按下下降键直至达到所需的检查床高度。

In the gantry operation interface, keep pressing the descending key until the required check bed height is reached.

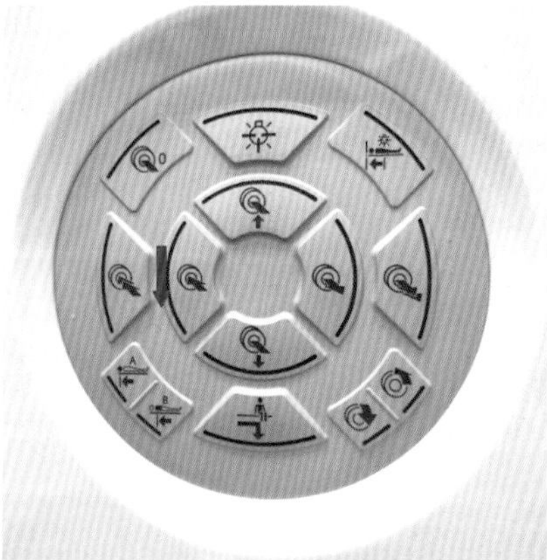

（2）仔细核对患者信息及固定模具，确认无误后进行摆位。

You must check the patient information and the fixed mould carefully, and then place the position after confirmation.

（3）打开激光灯。

Turn on the laser light.

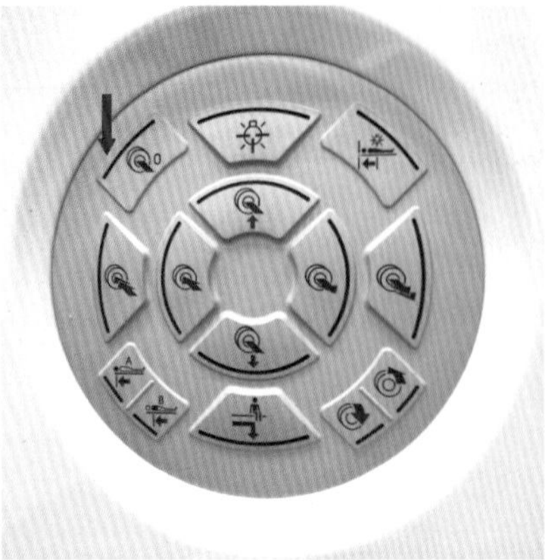

（4）摆放好患者定位使用的固定模具（体膜、负压袋、乳腺托架等）。

Lay out the fixed mould for the positioning of the patient （body membrane, negative pressure bag, breast bracket, etc.）

（5）将患者扶上床进行摆位，贴好铅点。

Put the patient into bed to place the position and stick the lead.

（6）设置扫描起点，使用水平移动键调整检查床的纵向位置。

Set the starting point of the scan, and use the move key to adjust the longitudinal position of the bed.

3 准备检查
(Prepare for check)

3.1 检查定位像参数（Check the positioning image parameters）

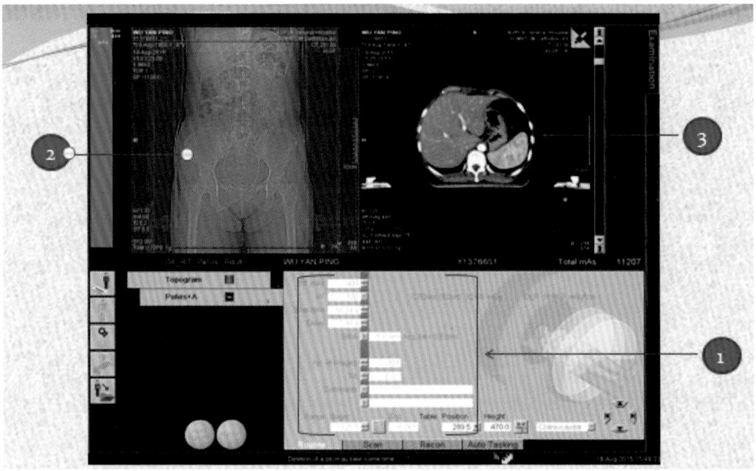

（1）在扫描次序列表中，选择定位像条目。

In the scan order list, select the positioning image entry.

（2）在常规参数卡中，检查定位像参数（管电流、管电压、层厚、球管位置）。

In the conventional parameter card, check the positioning image parameters （tube current, tube voltage, thickness, ball pipe position）

3.2　装载定位像（Load positioning image）

点击显示框下面的load键进行定位像采集，因患者身高及扫描范围的不同可以自由设置定位像长度，以达到扫描范围的要求。

Click the load button in below display box to collect positioning image, because of the patient's height and scan range, it is possible to set the positioning image length to reach the scanning range.

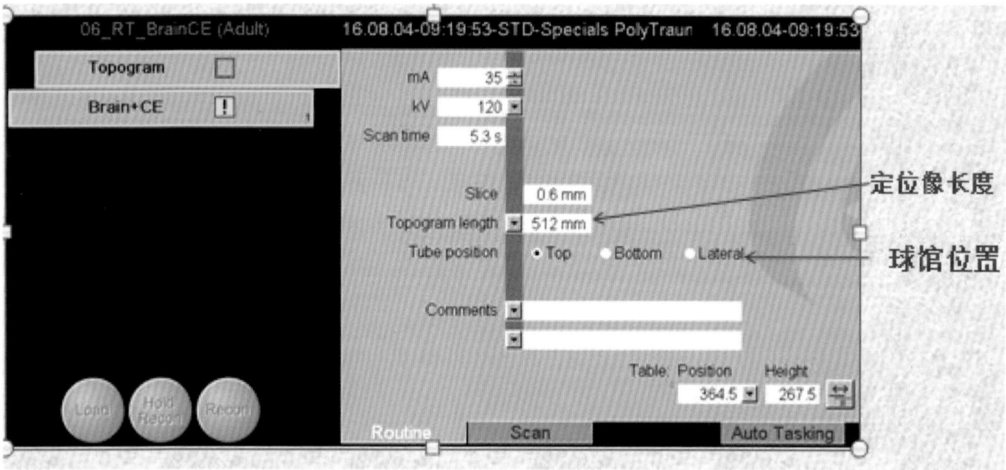

3.3　采集定位像（Collect positioning image）

（1）在控制盒上，按启动键。

Press the start button on the control box.

（2）定位像将显示在检查卡的左上像格中，如果已配置，则CARE profile显示在定位像的左侧。

The positioning image will be displayed on the top left image of the check card, and if configured, the CARE profile is displayed on the left side of the positioning image.

（3）后续条目的扫描范围和重建范围显示在定位像中。

The scan scope and reconstruction scope of subsequent entries are shown in the positioning image.

（4）未选中条目以灰色显示，选中条目通过以下颜色编码表示：

The unselected entry is shown in grey, and the selected item is encoded in the following color code:

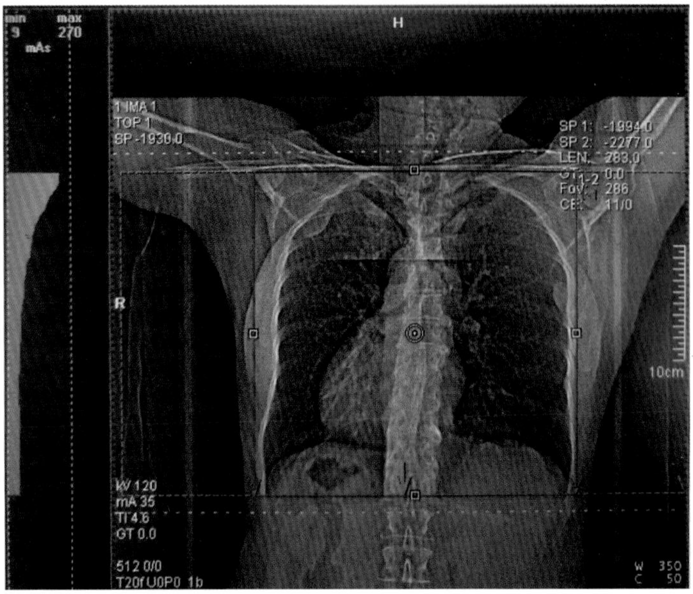

蓝色：扫描范围

Blue: scan range

紫红色：选中的重建范围

Burgundy: the selected redevelopment range

白色：未选中的重建范围

White: unselected redevelopment range

黄色：无效的扫描/重建范围

Yellow: invalid scan/reconstruct range

橙色：辐射区域

Orange: radiation area

3.4 高压注射器（High pressure syringe）

如果需要增强扫描，此时需要使用高压注射器，这是控制注射器的操作界面，需要设定注射造影剂的数量参数、流速、常规B筒。我们用生理盐水试针。

If you need to enhance the scanning, you need to use a high pressure syringe, which is the operation interface of the control syringe, and you need to set the number parameters of the injection contrast agent, the flow rate, routine for B tube. We often use a saline test needle.

（1）在这个界面就 可以设定相关参数，设定后按绿色箭头保存设定结果。

In this interface you can set the parameters, and then save the settings with pressing the green arrow。

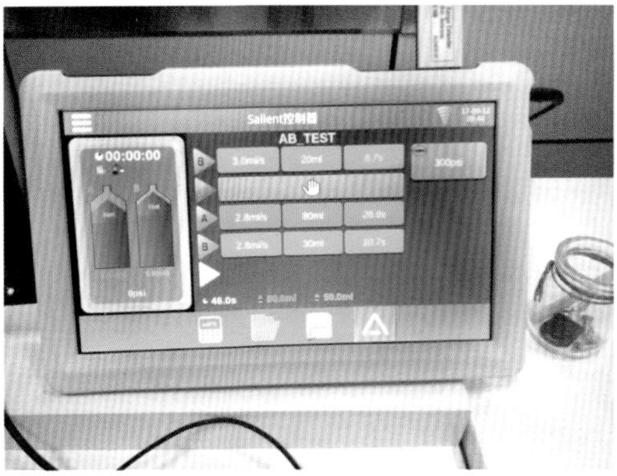

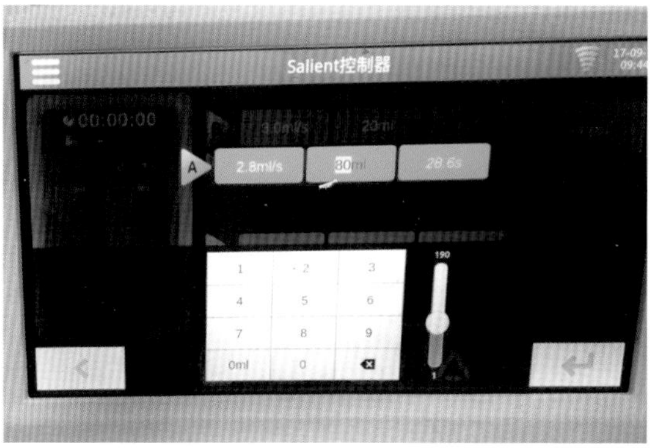

（2）点击绿色对号。

Click the green pair.

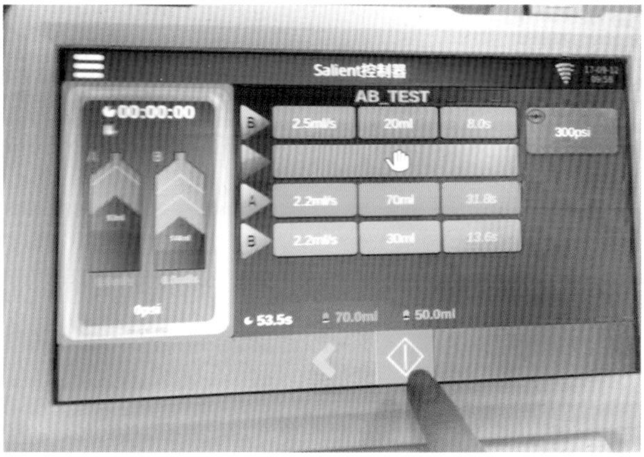

（3）这一步操作要和CT扫描的start键几乎同时进行，表示开始注射造影剂。

This operation is performed almost simultaneously with the start button of the CT scan, indicating that the injection contrast agent is started.

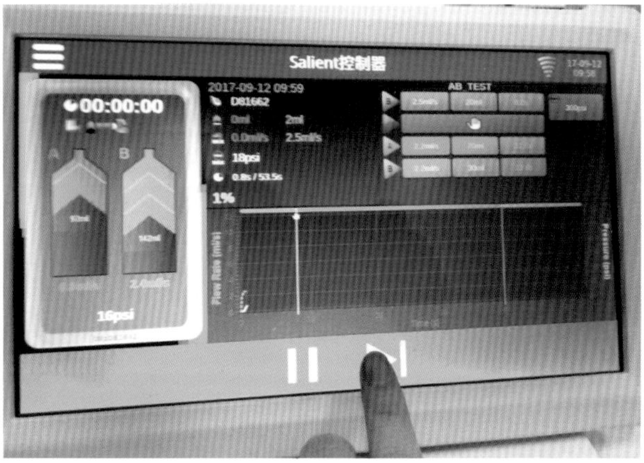

（4）扫描时时刻注意患者情况，有不适反应立即停止扫描。

Keep an eye on patient' s dynamics during the scanning process, and stop scanning immediately if there is any discomfort.

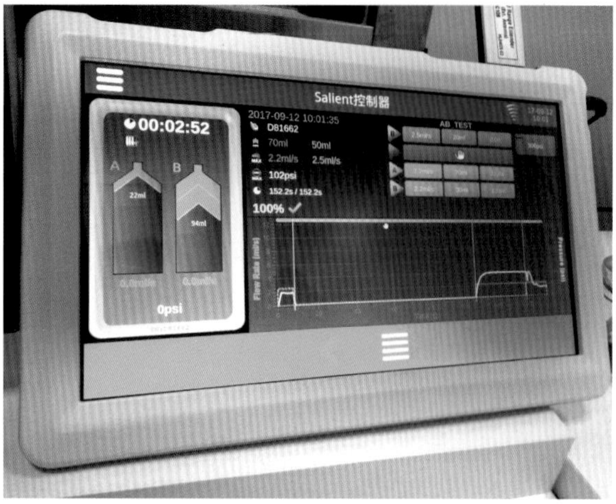

（5）做完一个病人后，点击返回键，进行下一个扫描。

After a patient is done, click the back button to perform the next scan.

4　相关页面操作

(Related page operation)

4.1　调整扫描范围大小（Adjust the scan scope size）

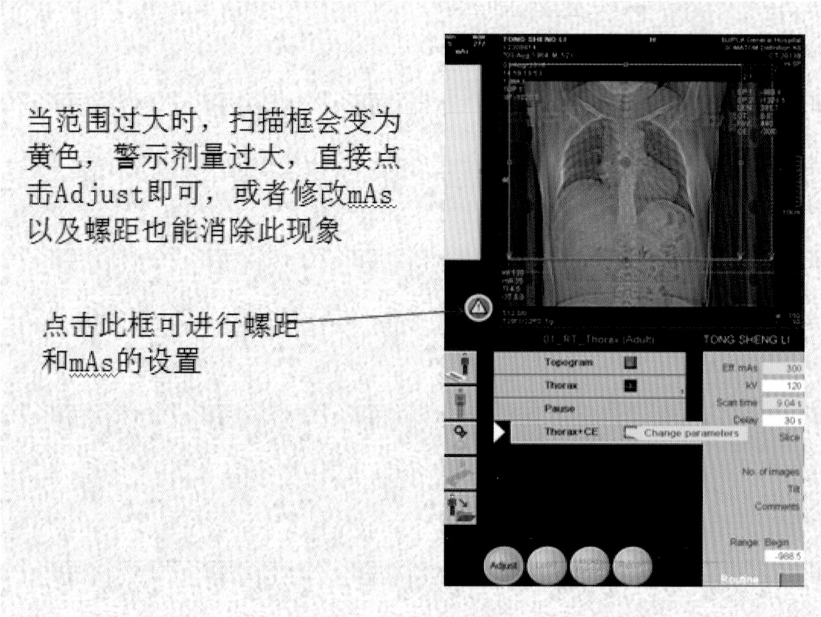

4.2　SCAN界面（SCAN interface）

· 剂量保护（Dose protection）

· 螺距（Pitch）

· 扫描方向（Scanning direction）
· 语音指令（Voice commands）

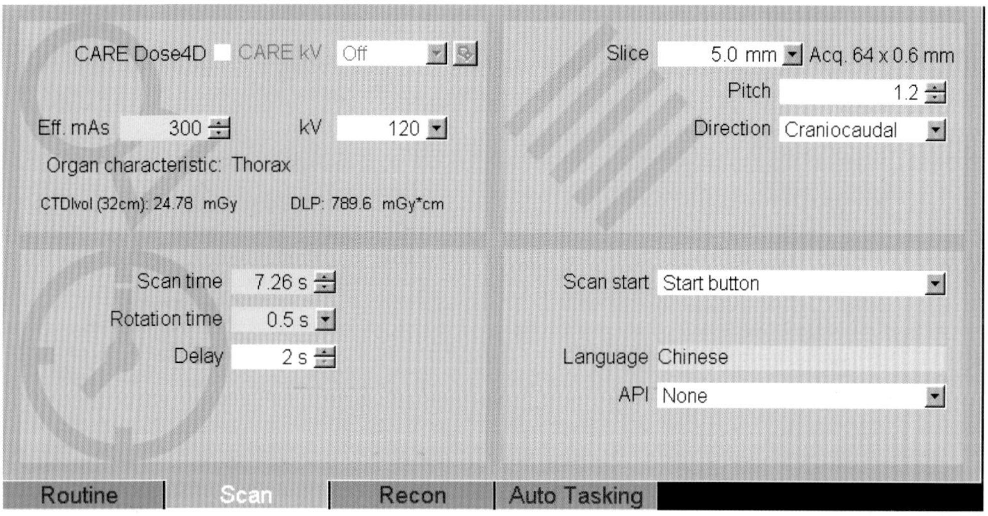

4.3 重建界面（Reconstruction of interface）

· 卷积（Convolution）
· 窗（Window）
· Fov
· 标注（Label）

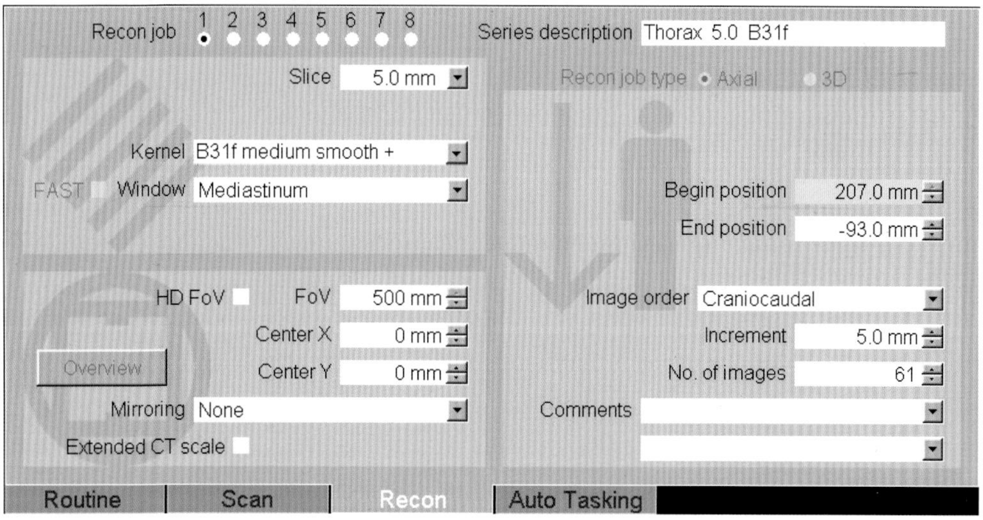

4.4 自动任务界面（Automatic task interface）

· 自动传输、打印（Automatic transmission and printing)

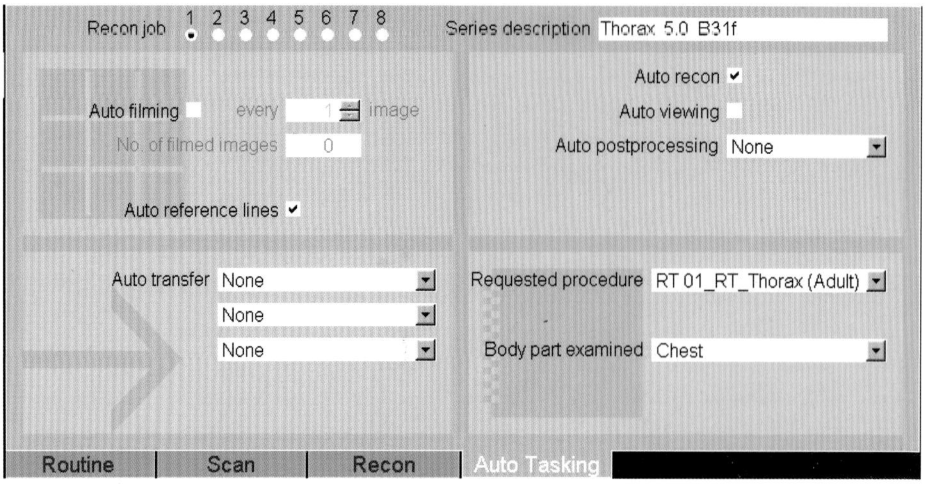

4.5 病人扫描结束后，将图像传输到医生要求的计划系统上。

(After the patient's scan, transmit the image to required planning system of the doctor.)

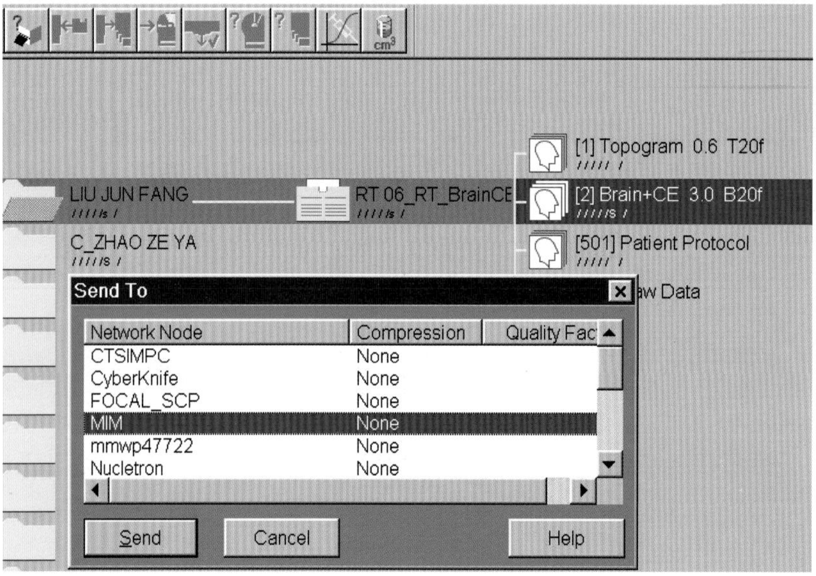

4.6 CT图像的后处理（Post-processing of CT images）

扫描完的病人图像有时需要后处理，在图像的层厚或者角度上进行重建，主要使用3D后处理软件。选择合适的层厚重建后，可以在filming进行CT胶片的打印。

The scanned patient's image sometimes needs to be reprocessed, reconstructed at the thickness or angle of the image, by mainly using 3D post-processing software. After reconstructing the appropriate layer, the CT film can be printed in filming.

4.7 如果需要刻盘，打开病人浏览器，点击transfer下的export选项即可。

(If you need a disk, open the client browser and click the export option in transfer.)

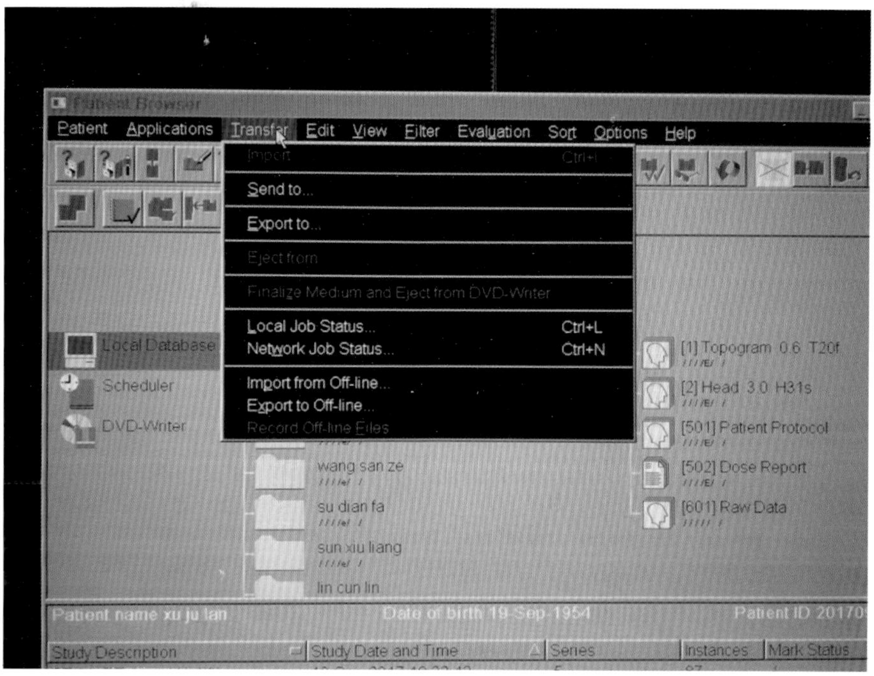

5 卸载病人

(Unload the patient)

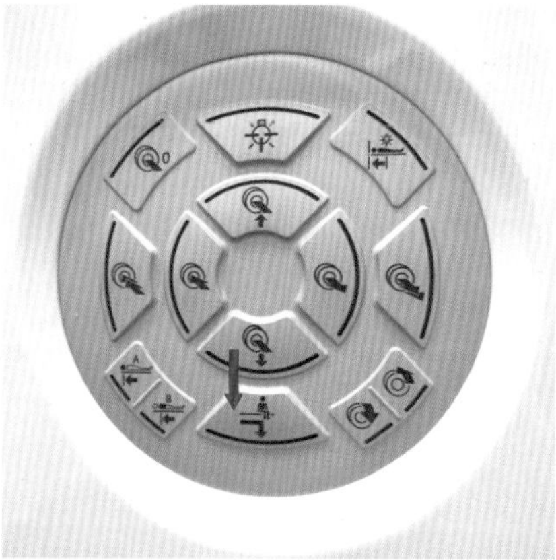

5.1 按下卸载键，将检查床从机架上移除。

(Press the unloading key to remove the bed from the gantry.)

5.2 进入机房将病人身上的模具取下，扶病人下床，检查结束。

(Enter the machine room to remove the mold from the patient, assist the patient to get out of bed, and all the operation is finished.)

6 关机流程

(The process of shutdown)

6.1 点击system选项下面的end选项。

Click the end option in the system option.

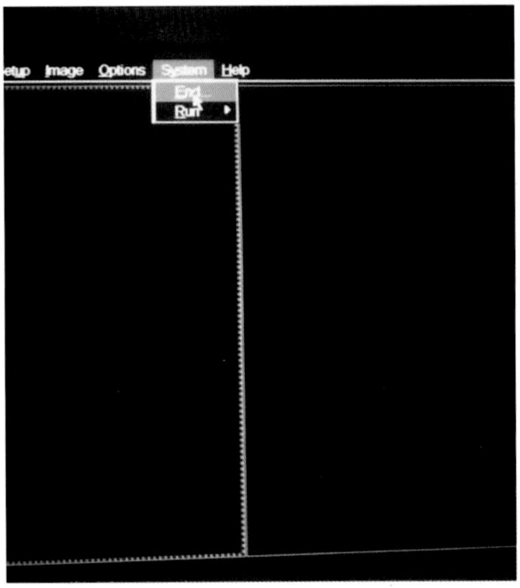

6.2 出现如下图所示的对话框，点击yes选项即可。

The dialog box appears as shown below, and click the yes.

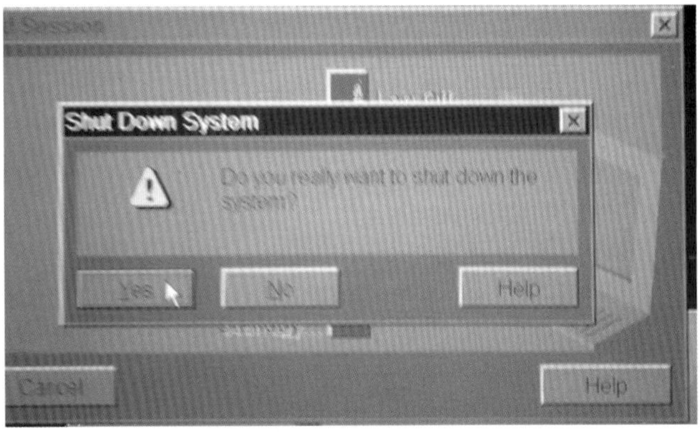

6.3 结束定位工作后，收拾工作台以及机房卫生，关好门窗水电。

After finishing positioning work, clean up the work table and the machine room sanitation, close the doors and windows and turn off water and electricity.

7 各部位扫描范围汇总

(The summary of scanning range of each part)

头部：头顶—锁骨头

Head: head - clavicular head

颈部：头顶—隆突（气管分叉）

Neck: head - juga （trachea bifurcation）

胸部：下颌骨—肝下缘（腰3/膈下）

Chest: lower jaw - liver lower margin （waist 3/ diaphragm）

腹部：隆突—腰4下缘（妇科至坐骨结节）

Abdomen: juga - waist 4 lower margin （gynecologic to ischial tuberosity）

盆腔：腰2上缘至会阴

Pelvic cavity: waist 2 upper margin - perineum

乳腺：下颌骨—膈下

Breast: lower jaw bone - diaphragm

四肢：手术全程—上下两个主要关节

Limb: surgery - the two main joints

第9节　碳离子放射治疗CT机质量保证和质量控制标准操作流程

Standard Operating Procedure for the QA and QC for CT Device in Carbon ion Radiotherapy

作者：康凯丽

1　CT设备每日开机自检

（CT equipment daily quality checkup）

开机画面结束后，机器进入检查界面，此时会自动弹出Checkup对话框，点击Checkup后操作面板上的Start键会闪烁，按下Start键进行自检。

注意：CT闲置4小时要做一次calibration。

At the end of the boot screen, the machine will enter the inspection interface. At this time, the Checkup dialog will be automatically popped up, and the Start button on the operating panel of the Checkup will blink, press the Start button for self-checkup.

Note: CT is idle for 4 hours for a calibration.

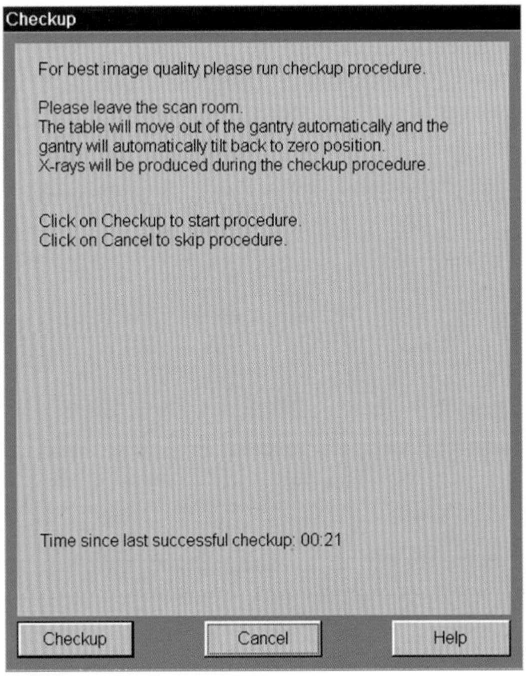

2 CT月检

(CT Monthly checkup)

(1) 激光定位灯（Laser positioning light）

如图所示，模体工具放置在激光标记处，通过升降床，核对所有激光线是否和标准模体标记线重合一致。

Set the module tool to the reference laser marks as shown in the figure, check whether all the laser lines coincide with the standard module marking line, using the lift bed.

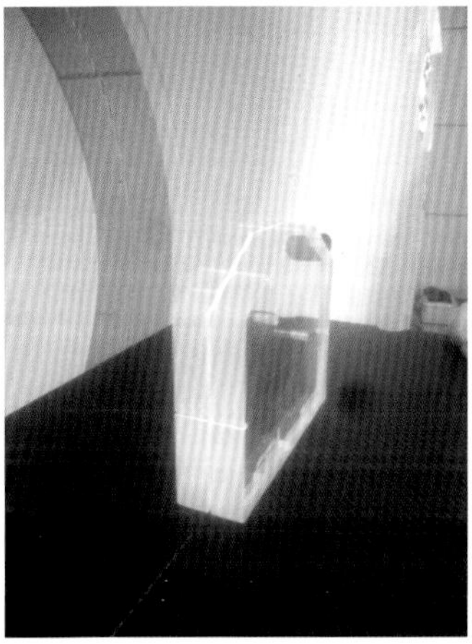

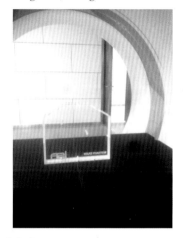

(2) 水模体*CT*值（The *CT* value of water module）

将水模体置于床头部，将床位置设置为激光标记体模的参考标记处，扫CT图像，测量*HU*值，和标准值对照。

Put the water module to the head part of the bed, set the bed position to the reference mark of the laser marker phantom, scan the CT image, measure the *HU* value, and control the standard value.

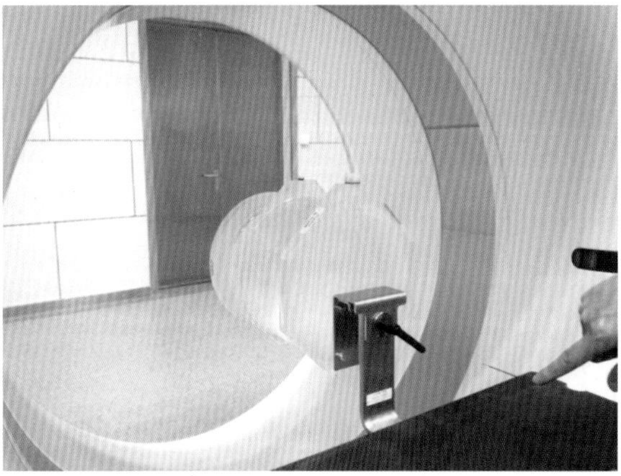

注意：要求水的平均值*CT*值正常波动范围不超过±3HU，空气的平均*CT*值不应超过±5HU。水模体内灌的水一定要新鲜或加有符合要求的防腐剂的蒸馏水，水中不能有

杂质，若灌注的水时间久了可能会有滋生菌类或藻类而影响检测的准确度，特别要避免产生气泡。

Note: the average *CT* value of normal fluctuation of water should not exceed plus or minus 3HU, and the average *CT* value of air should not exceed plus or minus 5HU. Water irrigated in the water phantom must be fresh or is distilled water which has preservatives that meet the requirements. There can be no impurities in water. Water kept over time may have fungus or algae and affect the accuracy of the detection. Avoid to produce bubbles especially.

（3）*CT*值

使用CT质控模体，模体最中心针管内为蒸馏水，其余固体为人体各脏器的组织等效材料，用于测定*CT*值误差是否在允许范围内。使用模体扫CT图像，并做数据分析，如下图：

Using the CT phantom equipment to check the behavior and quality. The core of the die body is distilled water. The rest of the solid is the tissue equivalent material of the organs of the body, which can be used to check whether the *CT* value error is within the allowable range. Use the phantom to scan the CT image, and do the data analysis, as shown in the picture below.

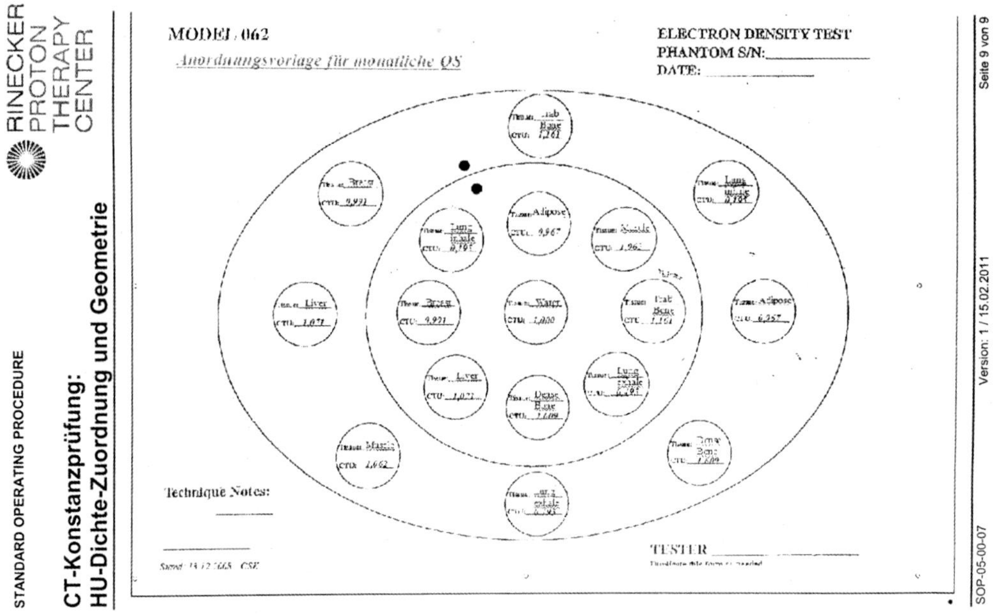

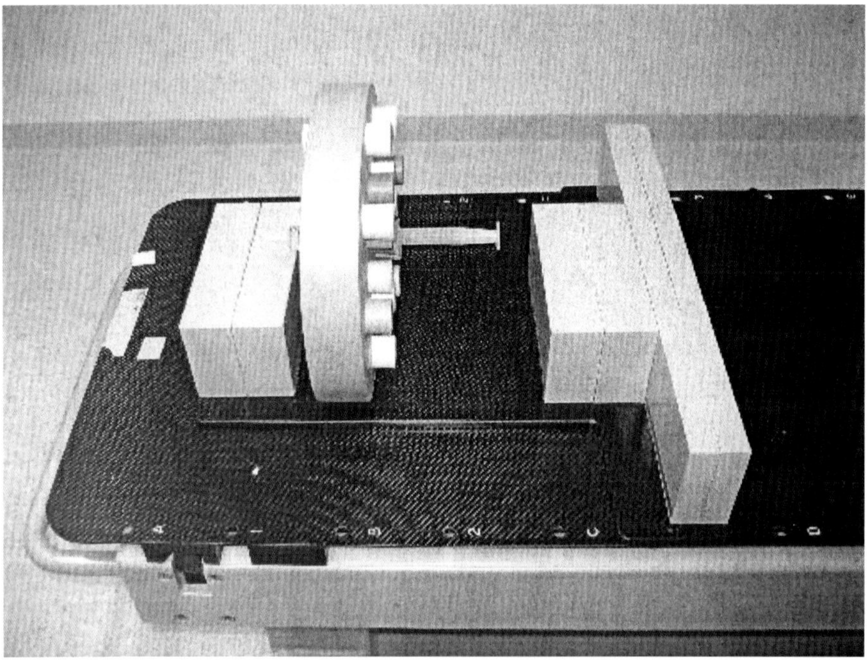

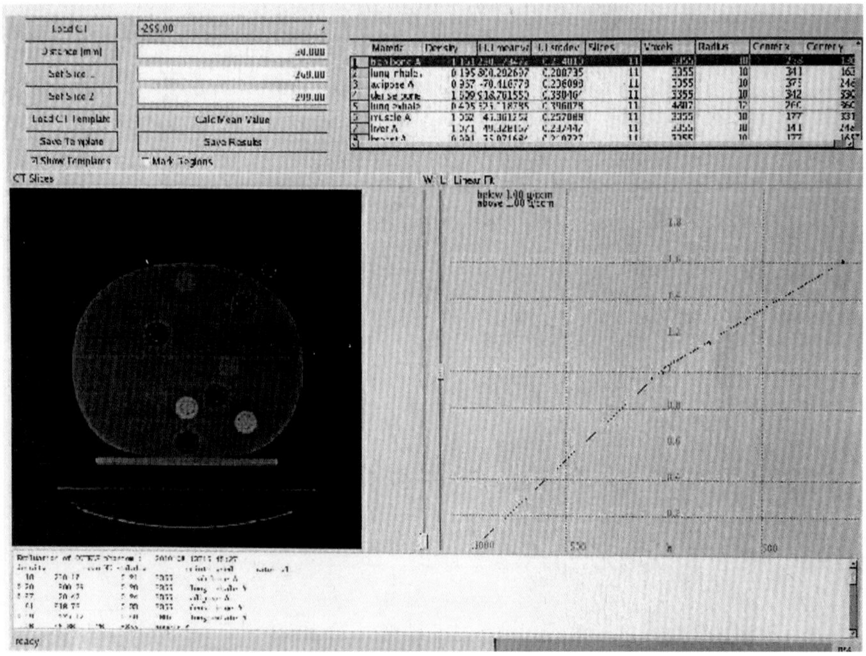
Load CT
Set Slice 1
Set Slice 2
Load CT Template
Save Template
Calc Mean Value
Save Results
CT Slices
Linear Fit
lung inhale
adipose A
muscle A
liver A
ready

第10节　碳离子放射治疗模拟定位激光灯标准操作流程
Standard Operating Procedure for Carbon Ion Radiotherapy Laser Light

作者：杨晓东　祁英　孟万斌　马霄云

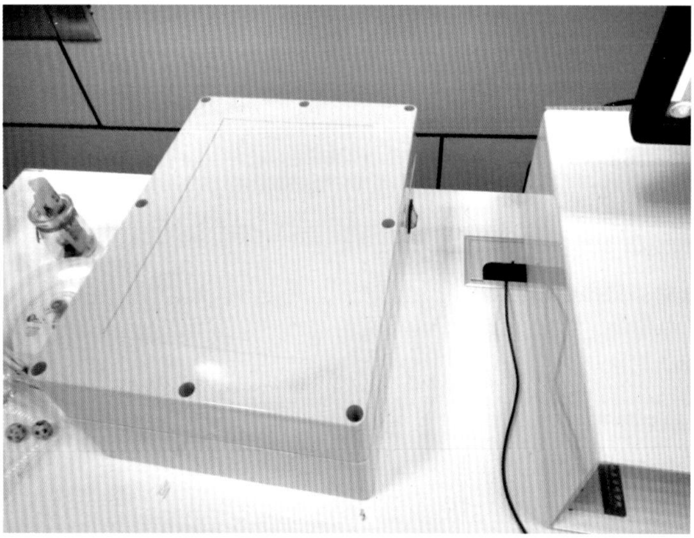

此图为激光灯的电源总控制盒子，每次使用之前摁开绿色按钮，接通激光灯电源。

This is the power supply control box of the laser light, press the green button every time before using, the power of the laser light is connected.

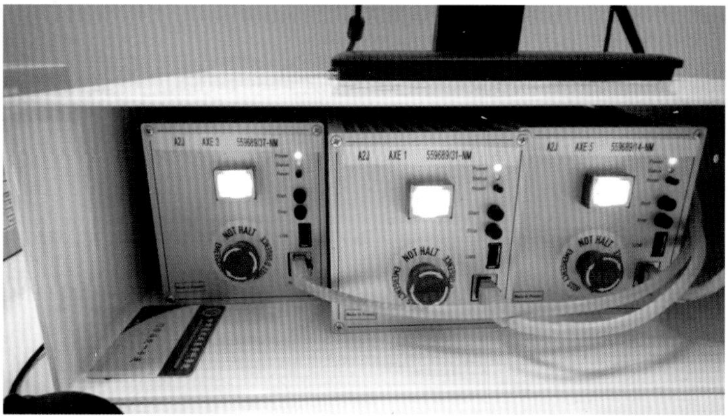

以上三个电源控制盒分别控制三个激光灯的电源，每次使用之前要摁开绿色的

power键，三个激光灯就都通电了。

These three power control boxes control the power supply of the three laser lights, and press the green power button every time before using, and the three laser lights are energized.

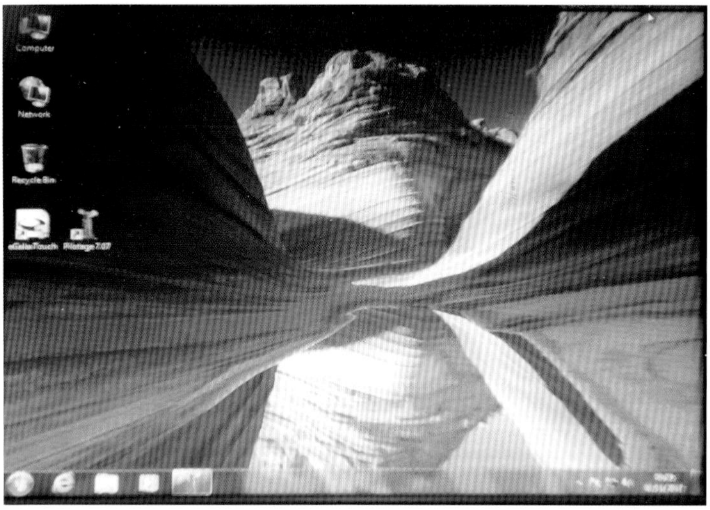

每次激光灯都需要复位到所需的位置，只需要点开控制激光灯的软件，激光灯就会自动复位到所需要的位置。

Reset the laser light to where we need, open the software that controls the laser light and it will automatically reset to where we need.

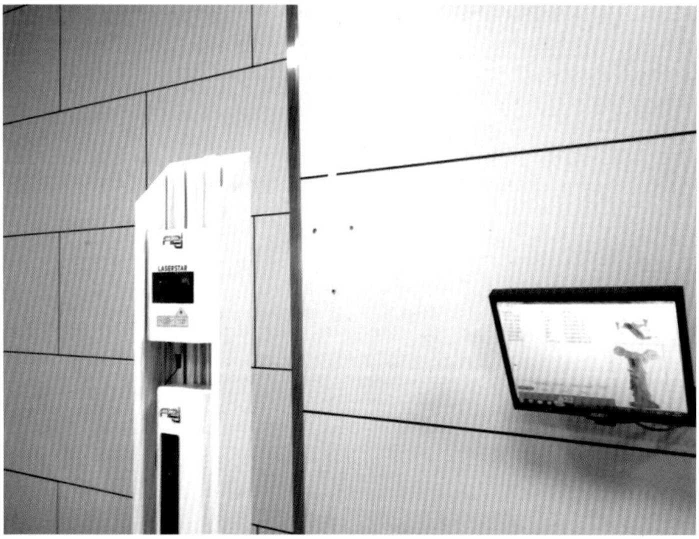

在工程师首次调整好激光灯的位置后，我们应该在墙上贴一条胶布，确定初始标准位置。此方法实用简单。在后期激光灯出现偏转时，通过里面的调节旋钮，将激光灯调整到初始画线的地方。

After the engineer has adjusted the position of the lamp for the first time, we should put a tape on the wall to determine the initial standard position. This method is practical and simple.

When the laser light deflects in the later stage, through the adjustment knob inside, we can adjust the laser light to the place where we drew the line.

关闭激光灯时要按一定的顺序进行，先关闭控制软件，然后关闭电脑、关闭控制电源的绿色按钮。

There must also be a certain order in the closure of the laser light. Turn off the control software firstly and turn off the computer. Then turn off the green button that controls the power supply.

注意：激光灯对人体眼睛会有伤害，在使用过程中一定要避免激光灯射入眼睛。

Note: The laser light will damage our eyes, and we must avoid the light bulb coming into our eyes during the process.

第11节 碳离子放射治疗恒温水箱标准操作流程
Standard Operating Procedure for Carbon Ion Rodiotherapy of Thermostatic Water Tank

作者：孟莉 孙洁仁 祁英 孟万斌 马霄云

放疗体位固定装置是放疗日常工作中的一个重要工具，在模拟定位和放疗摆位中有着重要作用；体位固定装置的应用显著提高了体位固定的重复性，对减少摆位误差、提高治疗精度有重要意义。热塑膜是常见体位固定装置其中之一，而恒温水箱是使用热塑膜的必需辅助设备。建立电热恒温水箱的标准操作规程，规范操作步骤，目的是延长设备使用寿命、确保工作顺利进行、保障操作人员人身安全和设备安全。

Radiotherapy immobilization fixation device is an important tool in the daily work of radiotherapy immobilization, and plays an important role in the simulation positioning and radiotherapy setting. The application of immobilization device significantly improves the immobilization repeatability, which is of great significance to reduce the setting error and improve the treatment accuracy.Thermoplastic mask is one of the most common immobilization devices, and thermostatic water tanks are necessary aids for the use of thermoplastic mask. Establish the thermostatic water tank's standard operating procedures, standard operation steps, in order to prolong the service life of equipment, ensure the work smoothly go on, guarantee staff personal safety and equipment safety.

1 将恒温水箱放在固定平台上，轻摇检查并确保其稳定性。

(Put the thermostatic water tank on the fixed platform, swipe gently to check and ensure its stability.)

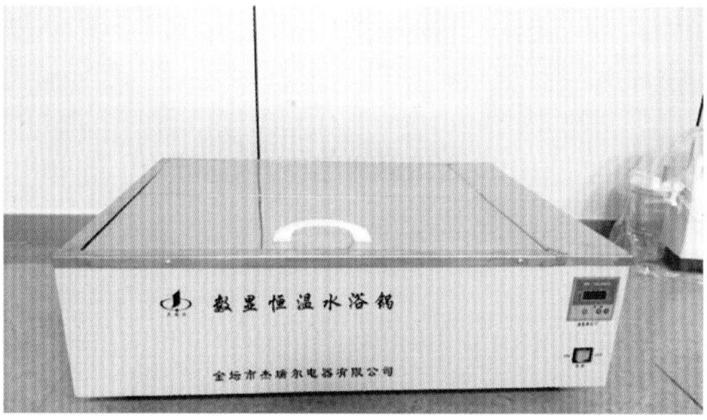

2　先将排水口开关关闭，防止有水从排水口漏出，再将水注入水箱内。

(First close drain switch to prevent water leakage from the drain, then inject water into the tank.)

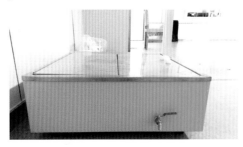

3　将按钮调至OFF，接通电源。

(Turn the button to OFF and turn on the power.)

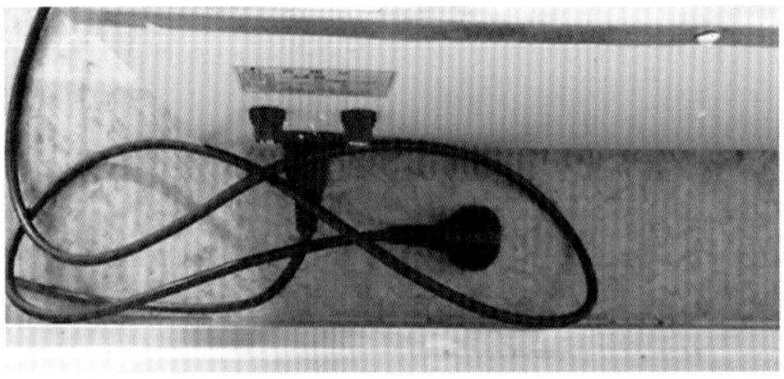

4　设定温度，一般为70 ℃。先按温度仪的功能键“SET”进入温度设定状态，SL设定显示灯亮，再按移位键配合加键“△”或减键“▽”，设定结束，按功能键“SET”确认。

(Set the temperature, usually 70 ℃. Press the function key “SET” of the thermometer to enter the temperature setting state. The SL setting indicator light will be on. Press the shift key together with the plus key “△” or the minus key “▽” to end the setting. Press the SET key to confirm.)

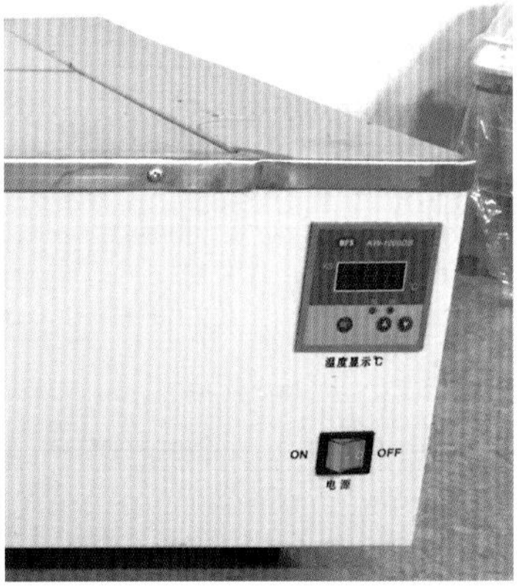

5 将开关按钮调至ON，水箱开始加热，水温逐渐升高，直至达到设定温度。

(Turn the button to ON, the thermostatic water tank starts to be heated up, and the water temperature gradually rises until the set temperature is reached.)

6 水温恒定后即可使用。

(Use it when the water temperature is constant.)

7 工作结束后，关闭电源。

(After work, turn off the power.)

8 定期加水，防止干烧。若使用自来水，应定期清洗。

(Regularly add water to prevent dry burning. If tap water is used, it should be cleaned periodically.)

第12节　碳离子放射治疗患者转移至治疗室标准操作流程
Standard Operating Procedure for Transporting Patients to the Treatment Room in Carbon Ion Radiotherapy

作者：李文祺　陈东基　祁英　孟万斌　马霄云

1　患者在准备间，在治疗车上将病人体位按治疗要求准备好。

（Put the patient on the transporter in the preparation room according to the treatment requirements.）

2　两名技师抓住转运车，从患者准备间推送至治疗室。

（Two technicians push the transporter from the preparation room to the treatment room.）

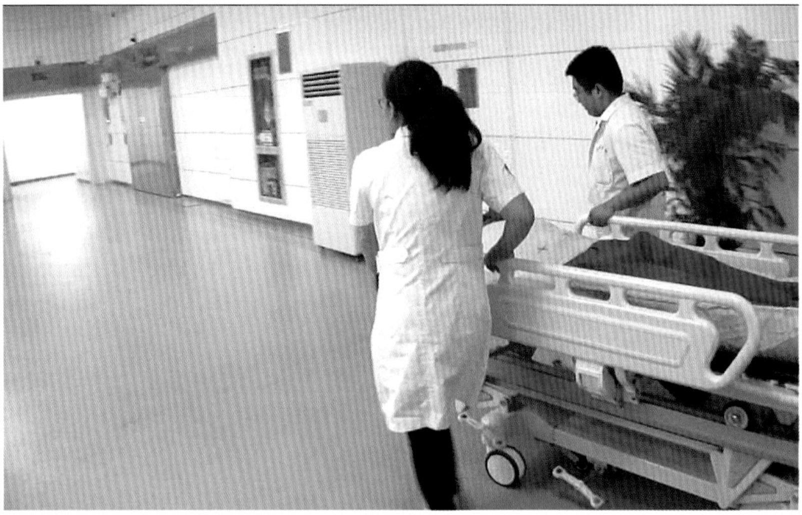

3　进入治疗室后，转动转运车至合适角度，与治疗床平行。

（After entering the treatment room, turn the transporter until parallel to the treatment bed.）

4　在治疗床上安装固定架，并插入转运板。

（Install the holder in the treatment bed and insert the transfer plate.）

5 调整治疗床和转运车到同一高度。

(Adjust the treatment bed and transporter to the same height.)

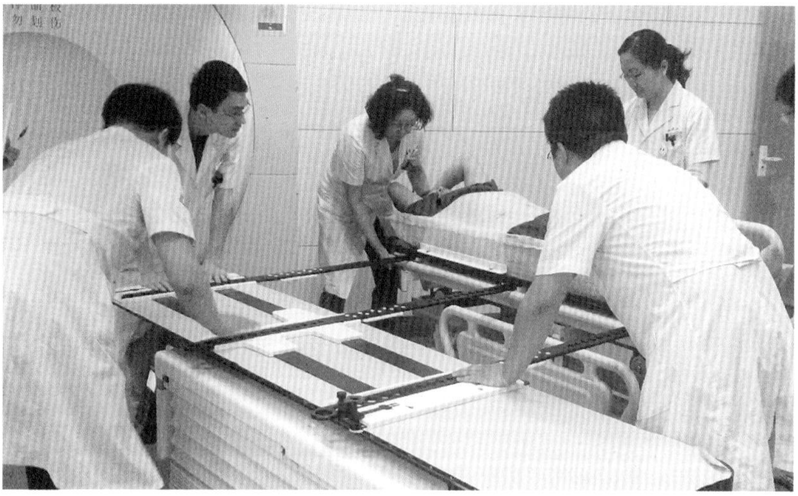

6 推转运车，令转运板完全插入转运车。

(Push the transporter, so that the transfer plate is fully inserted into the transporter.)

7 解开转运车的固定卡扣，推动病人和真空袋一起到治疗床上。

(Unlock the transporter's fixed catch, push the patient and vacuum bag to the treatment bed.)

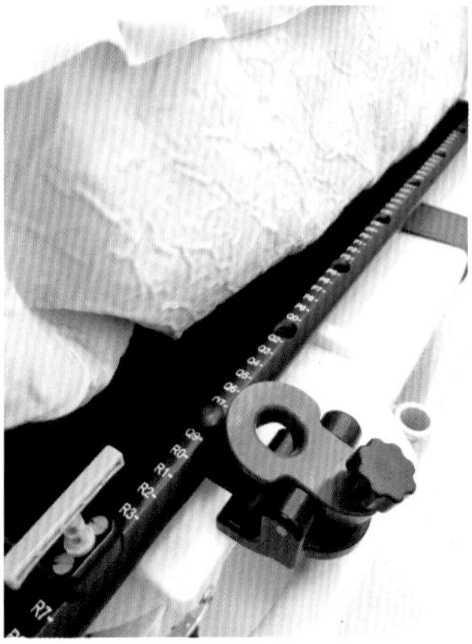

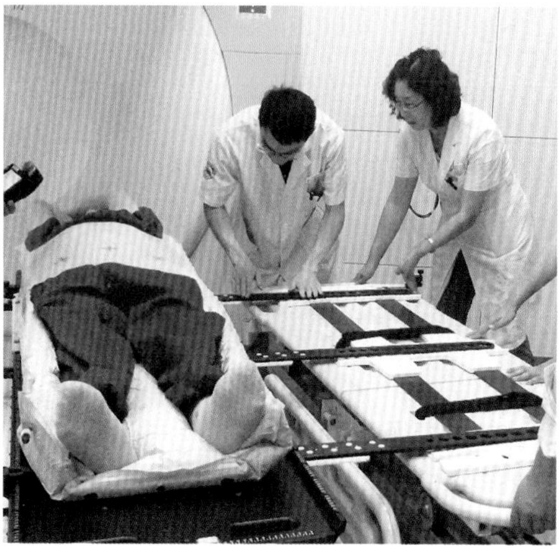

8 推开转运车，取出转运板。

(Push the transporter and remove the transfer plate.)

9　拧紧治疗床上固定卡扣。

（Closed the bed with a fixed catch.）

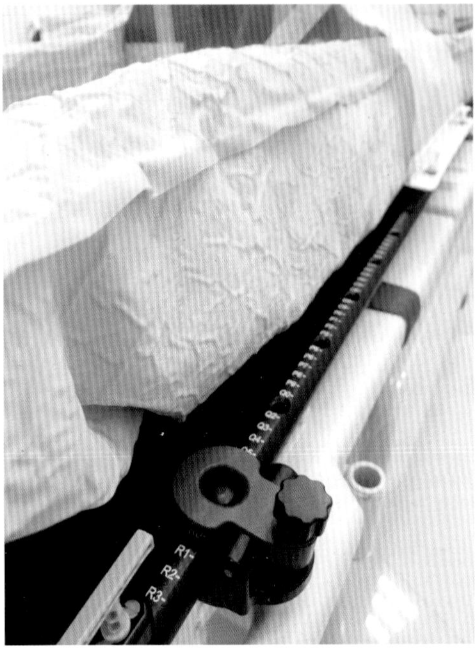

10　将转运车推至治疗室迷路走廊备用。

（Move the transporter out to the corridor of treatment room for the future use.）

第13节　碳离子放射治疗真空负压袋体位固定标准操作流程
Standard Operating Procedure for Vacuum Negative Pressure Bag Immobilization of Carbon Ion Radiotherapy

作者：孟莉　孙洁仁　祁英　孟万斌　马霄云

1　将Lok-Bar卡条固定于转运板上合适的位置
(Secure the Lok-Bar card in place on the transport plate)

我院目前所使用的负压袋为CIVCO提供的尺寸为80 cm×200 cm、内部由小的聚苯乙烯珠填充的专用负压袋。由于抽真空时负压袋会有一定程度的收缩，经反复试验，两Lok-Bar卡条间距约为190 cm（即两Lok-Bar卡条间距在等于负压袋长度后缩进两个转运板插孔）较为合适。

Negative pressure bag from CIVCO used in our hospital currently is size 80 cm× 200 cm, filled with the small polystyrene beads inside special negative pressure bag. Because the vacuum negative pressure bag will have a certain degree of contraction, after trial and error, two article Lok - Bar card distance is about 190 cm（That is, the spacing between the two Lok-Bar clamps is equal to the length of the negative pressure bag and then retracts into the two transport plate jacks） is more appropriate.

2　将真空垫平铺于转运板上
(Tilt the vacuum negative pressure bag on the transfer board)

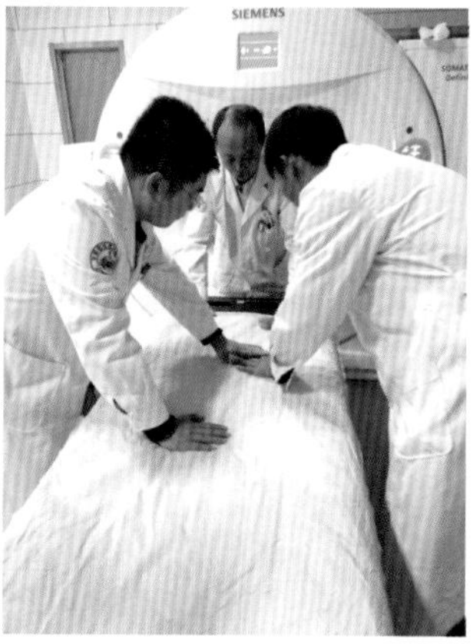

3　用卡条将负压袋固定

(Fix the vacuum bag with the clamps)

先用Lok-Bar固定负压袋一头，将负压袋另一头稍微收缩抚平再用另一个Lok-Bar固定。

First fix negative pressure bag one end with Lok-Bar,squeeze the other end of the vacuum bag a little and flatten it with another Lok-Bar.

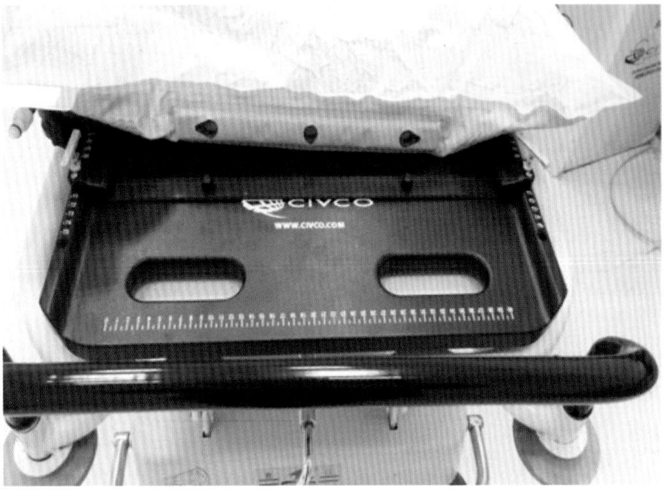

4　放置头枕

(Place the pillow)

于负压袋前端中间位置剖坑放置合适型号的头枕。

Place appropriate type of pillow in the negative pressure bag in the middle of the front position.

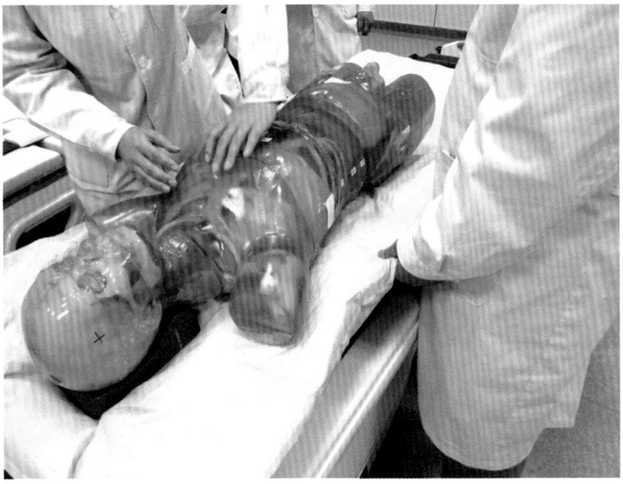

5 选择合适的体位

(Choose the right position)

让患者平躺（或俯卧）于真空垫内，双手交叉置于头顶。将患者置于负压袋正中间，卷起负压袋的边缘部分，紧贴于患者两侧，因为碳离子放射治疗的全身型负压袋比X射线放射治疗的负压袋长很多，所以目前的人员配置为4人协同完成。

The patient is supine (or prone) in the vacuum negative pressure bag, arms crossed on the top of the head. Place the patient in the middle of the negative pressure bag, roll up the edge of the negative pressure bag, close to the patient on both sides. Because the whole body negative pressure bag in carbon ion radiotherapy is much longer than that of the negative pressure bag in X-ray radiotherapy, the current work is done in coordination with 4 people.

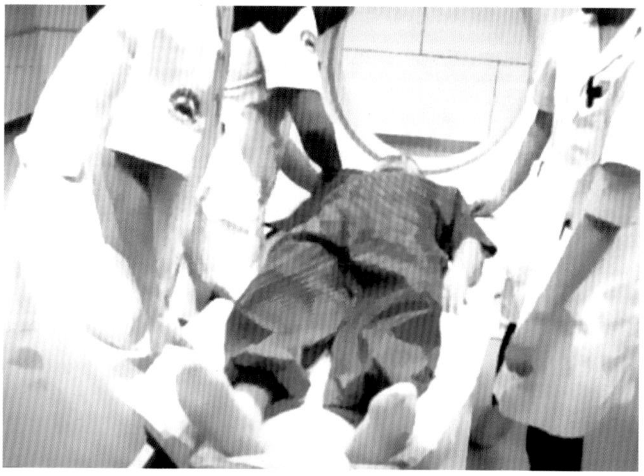

6 抽真空

(Vacuumize)

经反复试验，负压袋抽真空压力值为-0.08 MPa较为适宜。此阶段是最为关键的阶段，操作人员要仔细观察真空袋的硬化过程，确保真空袋每个部位的硬化都是我们预设的形状。

After trial and error, -0.08 MPa is more appropriate for negative pressure bag. This stage is the most critical stage. The operator should carefully observe the curing process of the vacuum bag to ensure that each part of the vacuum bag is hardened to our default shape.

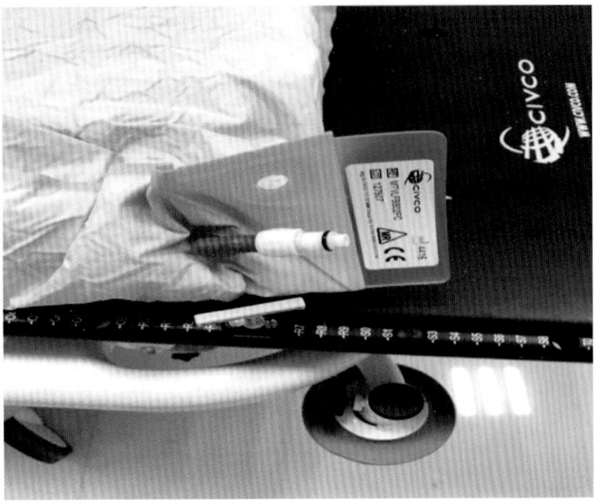

7 松开连接头，关闭真空泵，贴标签

(Release the connector, turn off the vacuum pump, attach a label)

将标签制成带有绑带的硬卡纸或是可直接粘于硬卡纸（或木牌，可重复使用）的胶贴，系于负压袋专用位置。

The labels shall be made with a bind tag cardboard paper, or can be directly on paper (or wooden, reusable) glue stick. Tie to the negative pressure bag special position.

患者负压袋专用标签				
患者姓名 Patient's name		性 别 Sex		患者专用二维码 Patient-specific QR code
患者ID Patient's ID		头枕号 Headrest model		
Lok-Bar位置 Lok-Bar position		负压袋压力值 Vacuum pressure value		
基准线位置 Baseline		特殊要求 special requirements		

8 从模拟定位床上取下放置于合适位置备用

(Remove from the simulated positioning bed, place to a suitable place for future use)

第14节　碳离子放射治疗真空泵标准操作流程
Standard Operating Procedure for Vacuum Pump in Carbon Ion Radiotherapy

作者：鲁会祥　祁英　孟万斌　马霄云

1　机器介绍
(Machine introduction)

真空泵是指利用机械、物理、化学或物理化学的方法对被抽容器进行抽气而获得真空的器件或设备。通俗来讲，真空泵是用各种方法在某一封闭空间中改善、产生和维持真空的装置。

The vacuum pump refers to a device or a equipment that using mechanical, physical, chemical or physicochemical methods of pumping the container to obtain the vacuum. In the popular sense, vacuum pumps are devices that use a variety of methods to improve, create, and maintain a vacuum in a confined space.

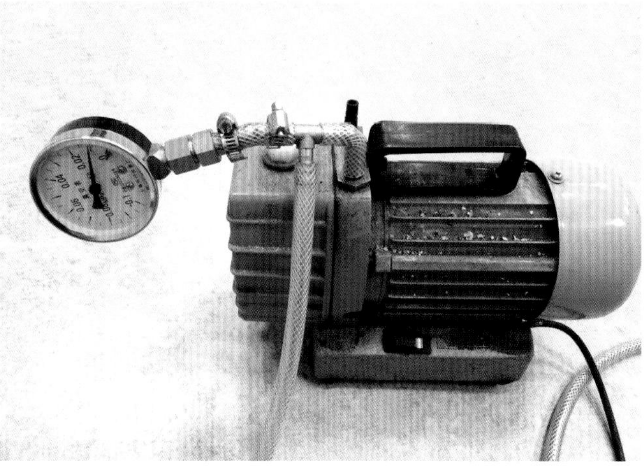

2　操作流程
(Operating procedures)

(1) 将新的负压袋平铺在床上，使袋中的颗粒四处均匀。

Put the new vacuum bag on the bed, make the particles in the bag evenly around.

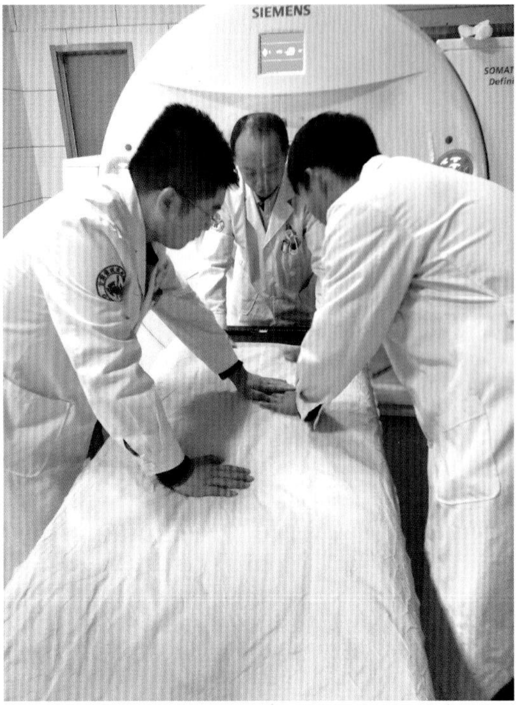

（2）根据病灶位置病人躺在负压袋上，利用负压袋对病人实施固定，负压袋初步塑型。

According to the location of the lesion, the patient lies on the vacuum bag, use vacuum bag to fix the patient, vacuum bag preliminary shapes.

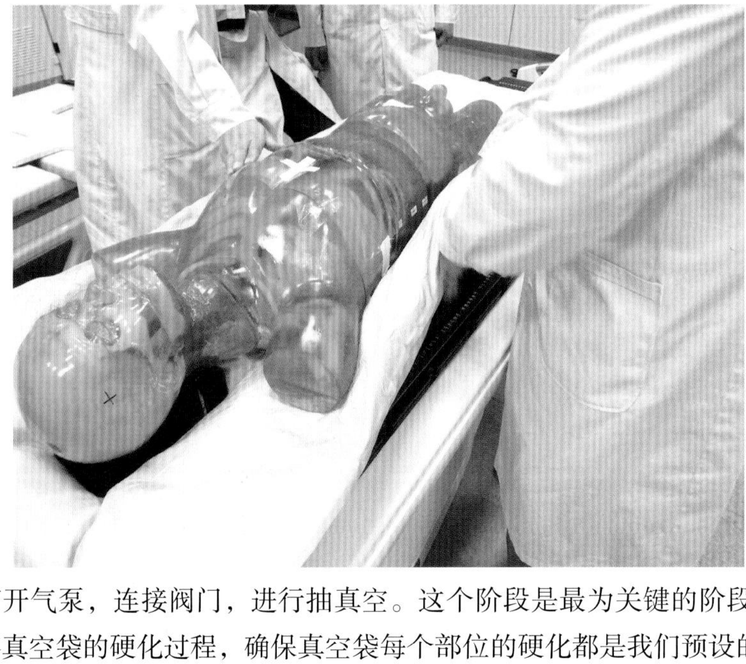

（3）打开气泵，连接阀门，进行抽真空。这个阶段是最为关键的阶段，操作人员要仔细观察真空袋的硬化过程，确保真空袋每个部位的硬化都是我们预设的形状。

Start the air pump, connect the valve to make vacuum. This stage is the most critical stage.

The operator should carefully observe the curing process of the vacuum bag to ensure that each part of the vacuum bag is hardened to our default shape.

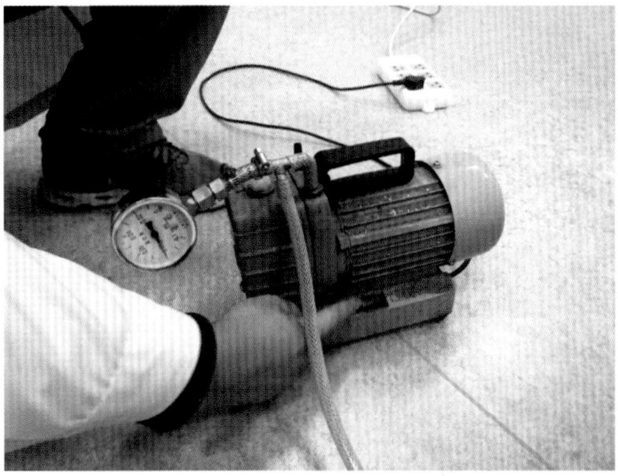

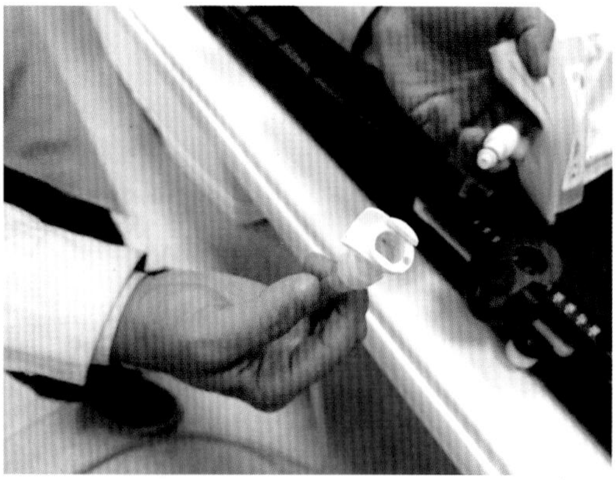

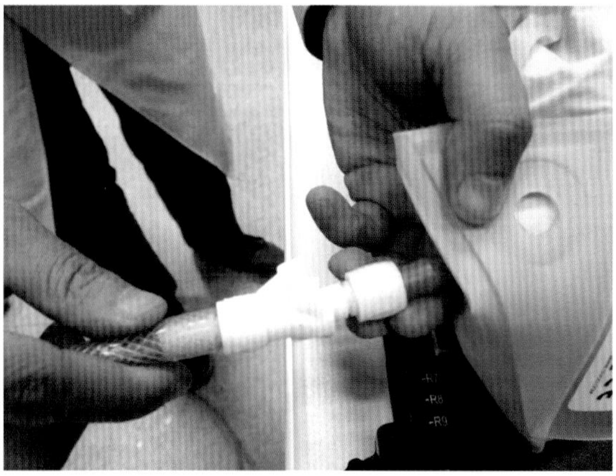

（4）一般情况当真空泵气压计显示到-0.08 MPa时负压袋塑型已完成。

Generally speaking, when the vacuum pump barometer shows －0.08 MPa, vacuum bag shape has been completed.

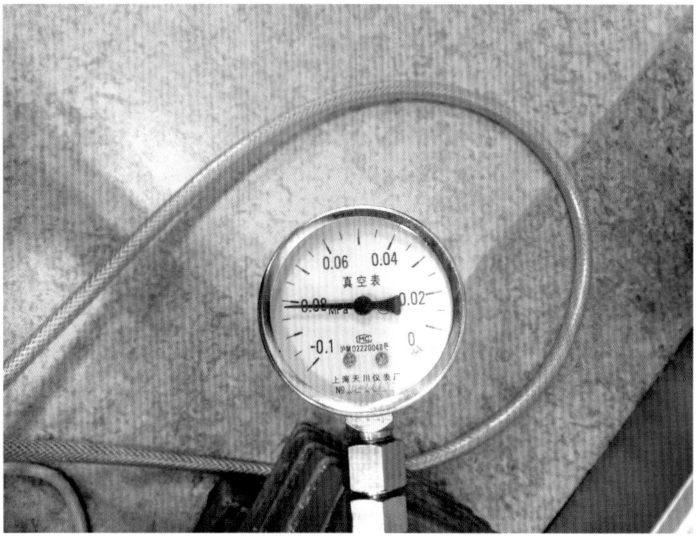

（5）关闭真空泵开关，撤去连接设备。

Turn off the vacuum pump switch and remove the connected equipment.

（6）将真空泵及连接设备放回原处。

Put the vacuum pump and connecting equipment back in place.

第15节　碳离子放射治疗患者位置确认标准操作流程
Standard Operating Procedure for Patient's Position Verification in Carbon Ion Radiotherapy

作者：朱芳芳　祁英　孟万斌　马霄云

患者位置确认在整个碳离子放射治疗过程中是极为关键的一步，可以说所有的体位精确固定都是为了最后更精确、更高效的位置确认做铺垫，所以患者的位置确认对医生以及技师的技术要求相对更严格，医生和技师必须具有扎实的影像解剖学基础以及丰富的患者位置确认经验。在摆位的过程中严格遵守摆位流程规范和ciGPS软件操作，做到精益求精、严把质量关。

Patient's position confirmation in the carbon ion radiotherapy is a crucial step in the process. We can say all the accurate immobilization is a groundwork for the final more accurate and more efficient immobilization, so the technical requirement for the doctors and technicians are relatively strict as for patient's position confirmation. Doctors and technicians must have a solid image anatomical basis, and rich experience in patient's position confirmed. In the process of positioning, strictly abide by the specification of positioning procedure and the operation of ciGPS software, and strive to keep improving and strict quality control.

下面，介绍患者位置确认的标准操作流程：

The standard operating procedure of the patient's positioning confirmation is described as follows:

1　前期准备
(Preliminary preparation)

1.1　患者摆位（Patient positioning）

DR设备是患者位置确认的主要硬件设备。如图，在患者的转运完成后，我们按照患者的摆位要求，将患者置于需治疗的等中心点处（图①），按患者治疗所需的要求，将DR设备控制至等中心点处（图②③④）。按照位置确认的要求，我们采取正交验证，即水平和垂直两个正交方向（图③④）。在控制DR的过程中，要密切注视DR臂与治疗床之间是否有碰床现象。

The DR device is the main hardware device for the patient's position confirmation. As shown in the figure, after the completion of the patient transfer, in accordance with the requirements for the patient's placement, put patients to treatment isocenter (figure ①). According to the requirement of the therapy, control the DR device to the isocenter (figure ②③④). According to the requirement of position confirmation, we adopt orthogonal verification, which is the horizontal and vertical orthogonal directions (figure ③④). During the control of DR, it is important to strictly observe whether there is a collision between DR arm and the treatment bed.

无论患者的病灶处于哪一部位，除了摆位过程存在差异，位置确认都是相同的，如图所示的是胸腹部患者的体位。

No matter where the lesion is located, except difference in the placement process, the position confirmation procedure is the same, as shown in the figure of the patient in the chest and abdomen.

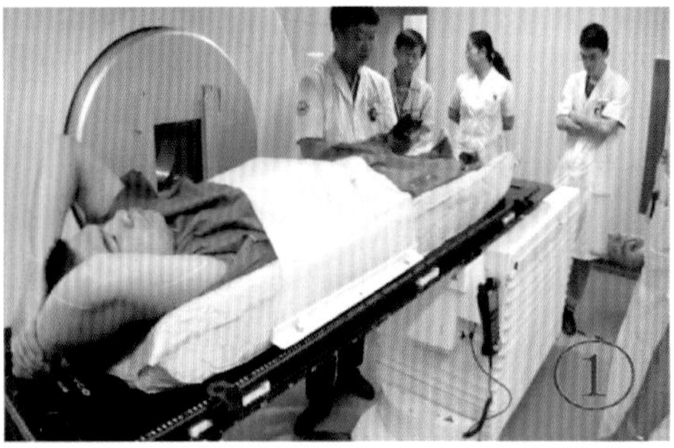

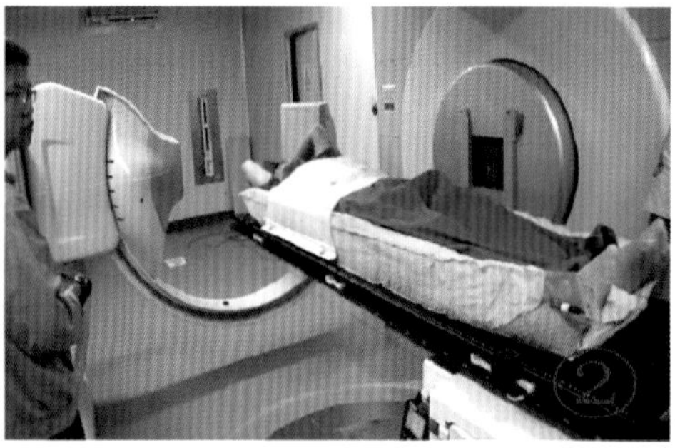

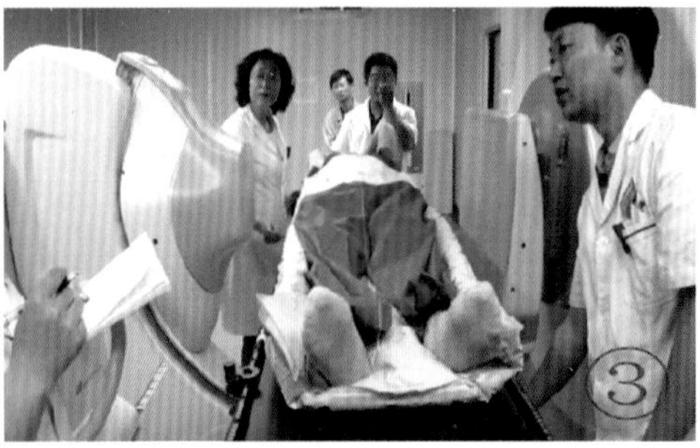

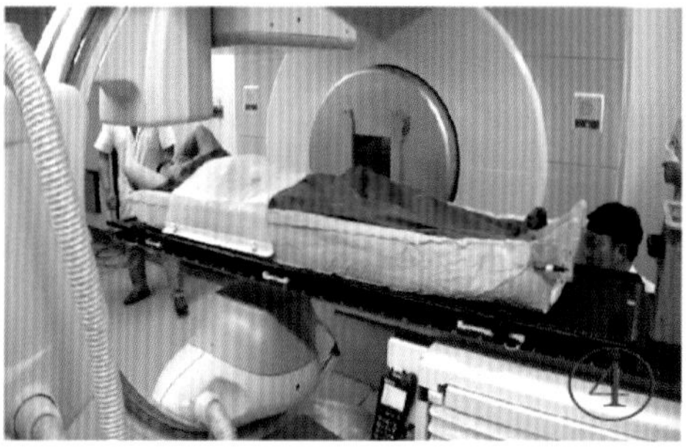

1.2　DR控制（DR Control）

可通过手柄对DR进行手动、自动、远程控制，也可根据不同的情况选择不同的模式进行控制。

The manual, automatic and remote control of DR can be done by the handle, and different modes can be used to control DR according to different situations.

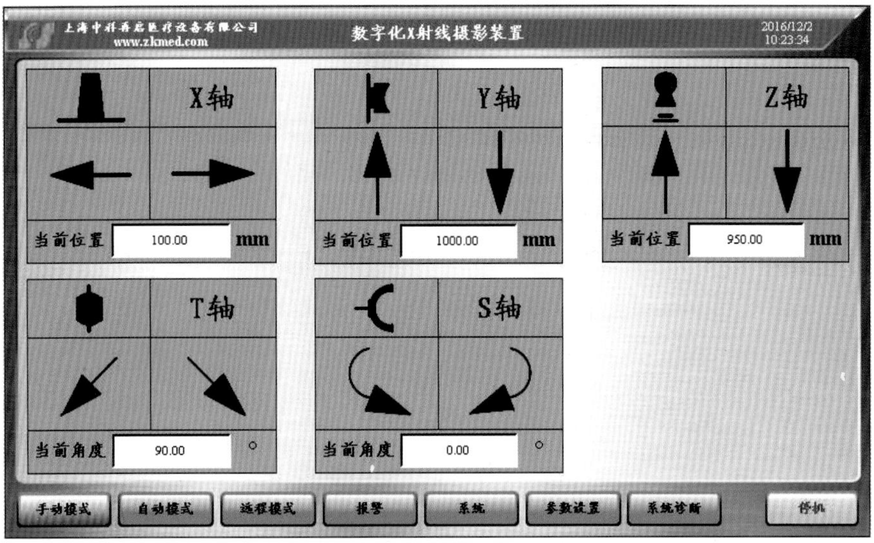

2　DR拍片

(DR Filming)

打开DR软件，进行登录，建立患者信息以及选取合适的体位，调试DR参数可按照如表所示厂家给出的经调试的参数进行设置。待所有的参数都准备好之后，可按曝光按钮（长按大约2～3 s）进行曝光拍片。如图为已经拍摄好的DR片。

Open DR software, log in, establish patient information and select the appropriate position, and debug DR parameters can be set according to the debugging parameters given by the manufacturer as shown in the table. After all the parameters are ready, press the exposure button (long press about 2 to 3s) for exposure. A filmed DR piece is shown in the figure.

距离1.8米时,柯尼卡板,东芝球管,CPI			距离1.2米时,柯尼卡板,东芝球管,CPI		
拍片部位	KV	MAS	拍片部位	KV	MAS
骨盆	84	36	骨盆	84	32
胸部(正)	105～112	12.5～16	胸部(正)	105～112	12.5～16
胸部(侧)	112～116	12.5～18	胸部(侧)	110～114	12.5～18
腹部	75	45	腹部	68	32
腰椎(正)	90	90	腰椎(正)	91	80
腰椎(侧)	105	90	腰椎(侧)	100	80
头颅(正)	80	20	头颅(正)	75	20
头颅(侧)	80	20	头颅(侧)	75	20

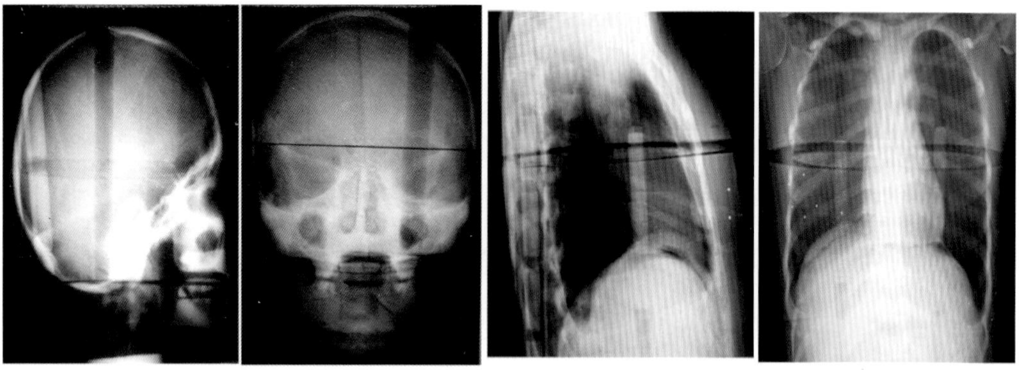

如图，曝光拍摄完成后，将已经拍摄好的DR图像按患者姓名传送至ciGPS。

As shown in the figure, after the exposure is completed, a filmed DR image will be sent to the ciGPS with the patient's name.

3 ciGPS

3.1 ciGPS软件介绍（ciGPS software introduction）

重离子摆位验证系统通过治疗前定位DR系统产生的患者DR影像与治疗计划CT数据的配准，计算治疗床的偏移量来引导患者摆位过程，确保治疗位置的准确性。

Registrate the patients DR image produced by the DR system before treatment and CT data of treatment plan in heavy ion beam position authentication system, calculate the offset of the bed to guide patients positioning process, to ensure the accuracy of the treatment position.

导入患者数据，数据包含CT图像、RTSS、RTPlan、两张DR图像和两张DRR图像。

Import patient data, which include CT images, RTSS, RTPlan, two DR images and two DRR images.

重置DRR图像至初始状态有手动配准和自动配准两种配准方式，配准结束后可以导出到ois系统。

With manual registration and automatic registration, the DRR image can be reset to the initial state and can be exported to the ois system after completion.

图像显示方式分为对比模式和重叠模式，提供了设置伪色彩功能，方便手动配准，提高配准的精确度。

The image display mode is divided into the comparison mode and the overlapping mode. There is the function of the fake color for convenient manual registration and the accuracy of the registration.

3.2 登录ciGPS（Login ciGPS）

运行程序，在登录界面输入正确的用户名和密码，点击login登录系统。

Run the program, enter the correct username and password in the login screen, and click login to login ciGPS system.

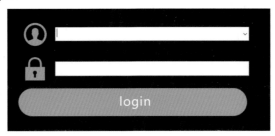

3.3 导入患者数据（Importing patient data）

如下图是对患者进行管理的主要功能按钮，ciGPS包含导入数据（Import）、导出数据（Export）和重置参数（Reset）3个功能。

The following figure is the main function button for managing the patient, and the ciGPS includes Import data (Import), Export data (Export) and Reset parameter (Reset)3 functions.

Import：用来导入患者数据

Reset：用来重置配准操作

Export：用来导出治疗床移动参数到OIS系统

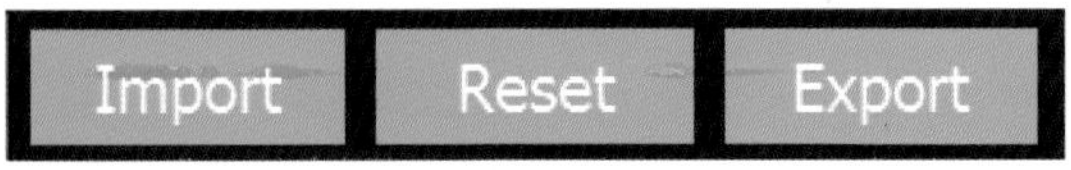

导入数据的操作步骤如下：

The steps to import data are as follows:

（1）点击Import打开导入界面

Click Import to open the Import interface

（2）点击Browse打开文件管理器

Click Browse to open the file manager

（3）选择要导入的数据所在文件夹

Select the folder where the data you want to import

（4）点击select folder按钮，数据路径显示在File Name内

Click the select folder button, and the data path is displayed in File Name

（5）点击Import按钮即可导入

Click Import button to Import

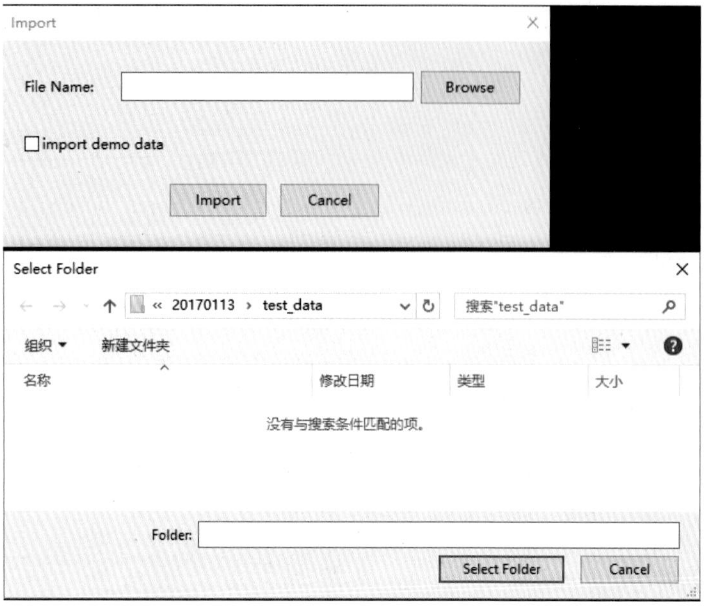

导入患者后可以在界面上方中间位置看到患者的基本信息，如图所示，基本信息包含：患者ID、患者姓名、患者性别和患者出生日期。

The patient's basic information can be seen in the middle of the interface after importing the patient, as shown in the figure, the basic information includes the patient is ID, the patient's name, the gender of the patient and the date of birth of the patient.

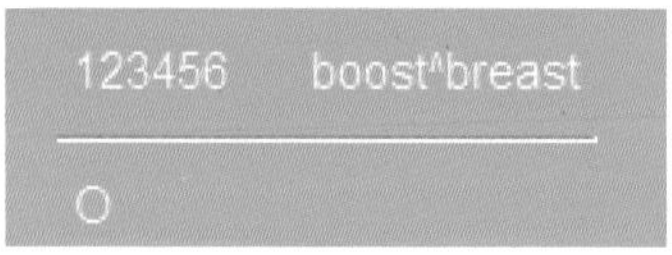

3.4 图像配准（Image registration）

ciGPS提供自动配准和手动配准两种方法。手动配准支持在x、y、z三个方向的平移以及绕着x、y、z三个轴的旋转。

ciGPS provides two methods of automatic and manual registration. Manual registration supports movement in the x, y and z plane and rotation around the axes of x, y.

3.4.1 手动配准（Manual registration）

Manual Registration是设置手动配准参数以及进行配准操作的控制面板。手动配准参数包括每次平移的距离和每次旋转的角度。

Manual Registration is the control panel that sets the manual registration parameter and the registration operation. Manual registration parameters include the distance of each translation and the angle of each rotation.

在step一栏可以设置手动配准时每一次操作调整的参数。在第一个输入框设置每一步平移操作时，治疗床平移的距离（mm为单位）；在第二个输入框设置每一步旋转操作时，治疗床旋转的角度（degree为单位）的参数。输入框编辑可只输入数字，也可以使用上下箭头调整数值。

In step column, you can set the parameters of each adjustment operation when using manual registration. In the first input box you can set treatment bed translation distance (mm as the unit) of every movement operation. In the second input box you can set treatment bed rotating angle (degree as unit parameters) of every rotation operation. The input box edits can enter the number just, or use up and down arrows to adjust the value.

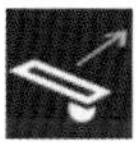	治疗床向右平移一段距离		治疗床向左平移一段距离
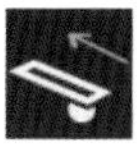	治疗床向后平移一段距离	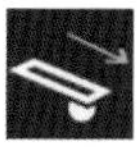	治疗床向前平移一段距离
	治疗床向上平移一段距离		治疗床向下平移一段距离
	治疗床绕着x轴逆时针旋转一定角度		治疗床绕着x轴顺时针旋转一定角度
	治疗床绕着y轴顺时针旋转一定角度		治疗床绕着y轴逆时针旋转一定角度
	治疗床绕着z轴逆时针旋转一定角度		治疗床绕着z轴顺时针旋转一定角度

3.4.2 自动配准（Auto Registration）

Auto Registration是自动配准区域，包含配准进度条、开始配准按钮和终止配准按钮，如图所示。

Auto Registration is an automatic Registration area, including registration progress bar, starting registration button and termination registration button, as shown in the figure.

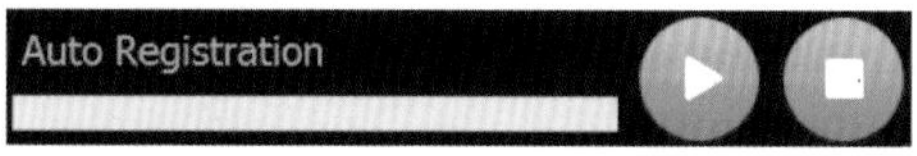

开启自动配准：Enable automatic registration

（1）点击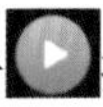按钮，开始配准

Click the 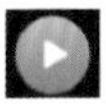 button to start registration

（2）DRR图像位置开始变动，偏移量和配准误差的值变化

The DRR image location starts to change, the offset and the registration error change

（3）配准完成，提示【Auto Registration completed!】

Registration complete, prompt【Auto Registration completed!】

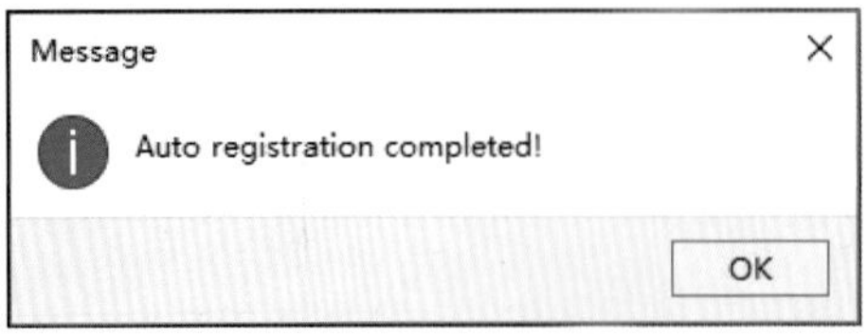

在配准的过程中，如出现故障如需重新摆位等情况，也可以终止自动配准：

In the process of registration, the automatic registration can also be terminated if the failure occurs such as the reposition of the position.

（1）点击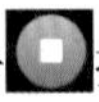按钮，提示【Auto Registration is in progress, are you sure to stop it?】

Click the 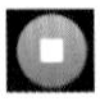 button, prompt【Auto Registration is in progress, are you sure to stop it?】

（2）点击OK，停止配准/点击Cancel，继续自动配准

Click OK, stop registration/click Cancel, and continue automatic registration.

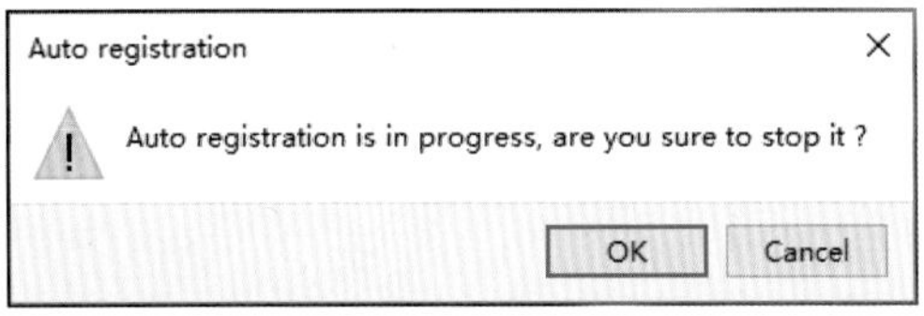

配准过程中：

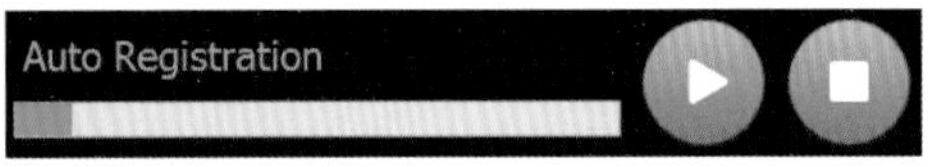

配准结束：

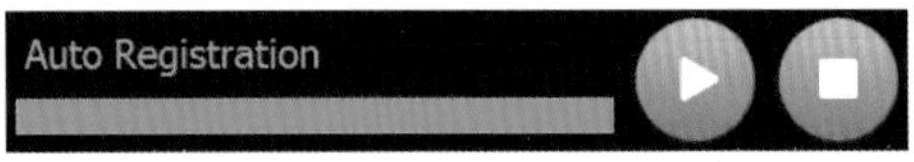

3.5　配准完成（Registration completed）

如果是手动配准，确保配准正确，主管医生已经确认签字后，方可执行治疗。但自动配准配准完成后必须进行移床操作，使患者处于正确的位置上。

If manual registration is used, and the registration is ensured to be correct, the competent doctor has confirmed and signed and the treatment can be performed. But the automatic registration of the registration be carried out on the bed, so that the patient is in the correct position.

3.5.1　治疗床偏移量显示（Treatment correction vector display）

Correction Vector区域显示治疗床的偏移量，如图所示。其中显示的信息为：

The Correction Vector area shows the offset of the treatment bed, as shown in the figure. The information shown here is:

（1）Lateral：侧面移动的距离和旋转的角度

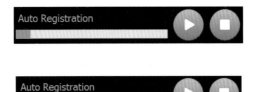

（2）Longitudinal：纵向移动的距离和旋转的角度

（3）Vertical：垂直移动的距离和旋转的角度

当使用者使用Manual Registration的平移和旋转按钮对图像进行平移、旋转时，偏移量会即时改变，并且与Step设置好的距离和角度一致。

When the user uses the Manual Registration translation and the rotation button to pan the image, the offset will change instantly, and the distance and angle of the Step will be aligned.

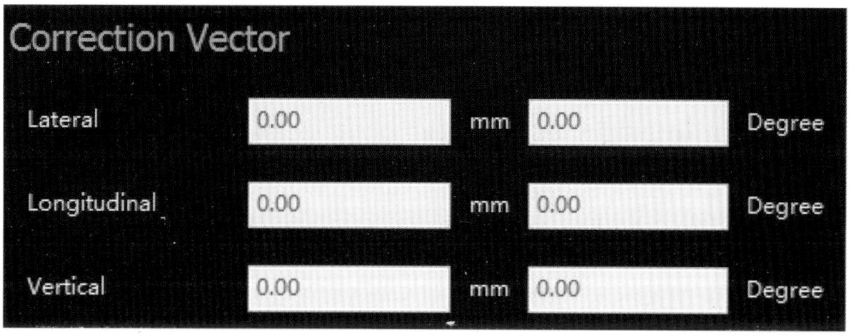

在Similaray Measurements显示配准误差，自动配准完成之后，在此区域显示配准的误差。

In the Similaray Measurements, the registration error is displayed and the registration error is displayed in this area after the automatic registration finished.

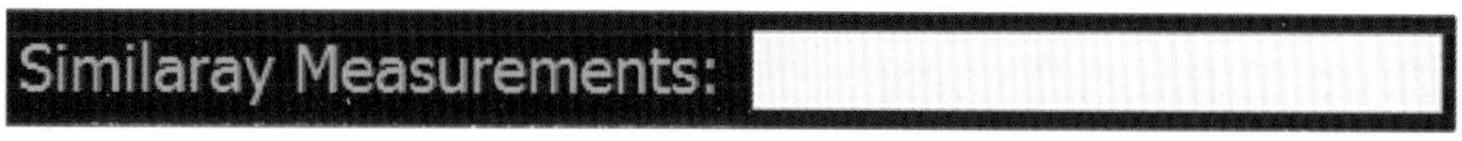

注意：只有自动配准显示误差，手动配准不显示误差。

Caution: The error is displayed in automatic registration mode only and not in manual registration mode.

在自动配准移床完成后，进行再拍片、再验证，看软件是否配准正确，一般情况下配准正确，如有配准错误出现，可以重新进行配准，直至配准正确，主管医生确认签字后，方可执行治疗。

In automatic registration after the completion of the moving bed, film, revalid again, to see whether the software registration is right. Under normal circumstances, the registration is correct, if there is any registration errors, registrate again, until the registration is right. The treatment can't be performed until the competent doctors confirmed and signed.

第16节 碳离子放射治疗患者准备间标准操作流程
Standard Operating Procedures for Patients Preparation Room in Carbon Ion Radiotherapy

作者：朱芳芳 祁英 孟万斌 马霄云

碳离子放射治疗患者准备间设计要合理，使用方便。按照碳离子放射治疗的要求结合重离子医院的实际情况，该准备间由两个部分组成。

The design of carbon ion radiotherapy patients preparation room should be reasonable and easy to use. According to the requirements of carbon ion radiotherapy and the actual situation of the heavy ion hospital, the preparation room is made up of two parts.

1 患者准备间

(Preparation room)

本院有两个患者准备间，男女各一间。两准备间相邻，处于整间准备间的最中央，四面的围墙由可拉伸的布帘组成。准备间内设有患者置衣架、放置私人物品的衣柜、可移动式台阶等，另外还设置了两间准备间通用的吊式可伸缩手柄，靠墙一侧设置扶手，便于在患者上下床时可双手握住吊式手柄或扶手，以便提高准备间患者的准备效率，预防坠床事件的发生。

There are two patients preparation rooms in our hospital, one for male patients and the other for female patients. They are adjacent and in the middle of the whole preparation room. At the same time, the surrounding walls are made up of stretchable curtains. There are patients coat hanger, chest for personal items, portable steps. Between the two are scalable general handle, and close the wall are handrail, so patients can hang the handle or grasp the handrail when get on and out the bed, in order to improve the efficiency of preparing between patients.

2 固定膜具放置架

(Immobilization equipment holder)

固定膜具放置架位于患者准备间的后方，紧贴墙面而设计，用以存放患者的固定膜具。在设计上与准备间相邻，方便取放，可在一定程度上提高准备工作效率。

下面介绍患者准备间的标准操作流程：

The immobilization equipment holder is located in the rear of the patient' s preparation room and designed close to the wall to hold the patient' s fixed immobilization. It is designed adjacent to the preparation room so it can be easy to use, to improve the preparation efficiency to a certain extent.

（1）患者信息登记（Patient information registration）

在进入准备间前，先依据患者的治疗申请单做相关的信息登记，按照治疗申请单的详细信息，确认患者所需的固定膜具，用二维码扫描仪进行逐一扫描，扫描完后再进行人工信息确认，务必保证信息与病人一致。

Before the patient enters the preparation room, according to the patient' s treatment application form, make the relevant information registration. According to the detailed information of the treatment application form, the immobilization equipment required by the patient is confirmed and the two dimensional code scanner is used to scan each one. After scanning, the information can be manual confirmed and the information must be consistent with the patient.

（2）更换病员服（Change of patient clothing）

待患者信息确认完毕后，找出患者专属的治疗病员服，因患者的治疗部位以及体型千差万别，务必保证病员服信息与患者一致。在更换病员服期间，要求一名行动敏捷、意识清醒、患者信任的家属陪同，不可太多，以免使准备间拥挤，造成不必要的麻烦。家属要协同摆位技师做好详细的解释和安抚工作，避免患者精神紧张。患者更换的衣服放置在置衣架上、衣柜内，切勿让家属自己保存，以免出现财产丢失等情况。

After the patient information is confirmed, find out the patient' s special suit. The location and size of the patient vary. Ensure that the patient' s clothing information is consistent with the patients. During the change of patient clothing, a family member who is alert, conscious and patient trust is required. The family members can' t be too many, so as not to make the preparation crowded and cause unnecessary trouble. The family members should coordinate with the technician to provide detailed explanation and reassurance so the patient isn' t scared. The replaced clothes are placed in a hanger or closet. Do not allow family members to save themselves, so as to avoid the loss of property.

（3）患者摆位（Patient positioning）

患者摆位是整个准备间最为关键的操作，我们可参照患者膜具制作过程进行摆位。头部、颈部膜具制作相同，可全部采用。胸腹部肿瘤患者的摆位相对复杂，下面就以胸腹部患者为例，做进一步讲解。

Patient positioning is the most critical operation in the whole preparation room. We can use the patient mask making procedure to position the patient. Because the head, head and neck thermoplastic mask making procedures are the same, we can adopt them. The positioning of the chest and abdomen tumor patients is relatively complex. The following is a case study of positioning of the chest and abdomen tumor patients.

①首先，将转运床的万向轮锁死，确保在各个方向上不能移动。按照患者治疗单信息，将SBRT转运板、Lok-Bar按参数设置好，务必保证参数设置正确。将患者的专属灰袋子按Lok-Bar卡扣位置固定于SBRT转运床板上以及专属头枕置于灰袋子头枕的专属位置。

First, lock the universal wheel of the transporters. Make sure you can't move it in every direction. According to the patient's treatment information, set the SBRT transport plate and Lok - Bar with parameters. Make sure the parameters are set correctly. Place the patient's exclusive gray bag on the SBRT transporter with the position of Lok - Bar buckle. Ensure that the dedicated pillow is placed in the dedicated position of the gray bag pillow.

②将台阶按患者习惯上床的方式置于患者习惯的位置，患者可在摆位技师的引导下上下台阶、上下治疗床。如需用到吊式手柄，也可在技师的指导下完成。且不可让患者及家属擅自行动。在整个摆位的过程中，摆位技师要时刻保持高度的警惕，以避免患者坠床等事件的发生。

Place the steps in the position according to the patient's go to bed habit. The patient can up and down stairs, get on and off the treatment bed with the guidance of the setting technician. If you need to use a sling handle, you can complete it under the guidance of the technician. And do not allow patients and their family members to act without authorization. During the whole patient positioning, the technician must be on high alert all the time. To avoid the occurrence of events such as falling from the bed.

③待患者成功固定于灰袋子之中后，再按照热塑膜的参数，将患者的热塑膜固定于SBRT板上。

After the patient is successfully fixed in the gray bag, according to the parameters of thermoplastic mask, fix the patient's thermoplastic mask on SBRT.

④为确保放射治疗的准确性、精确性，务必在以上操作完成后进行患者信息的再查对。包括患者姓名、性别、住院号、固定膜具信息、Lok-Bar、头枕的信息等。

To ensure the correctness and accuracy of radiotherapy, be sure to check the patient information again after the above operation being completed, which includes patient's name, gender and hospital number, information of immobilization, Lok-Bar, pillow information, etc.

第17节　碳离子放射治疗转运床标准操作流程
Standard Operating Procedure for Carbon Ion Therapy Trolley

作者：王开平　祁英　孟万斌　马霄云

1.将转运模块固定在转运车床面上。

Fix the transfer module on the trolley lathe.

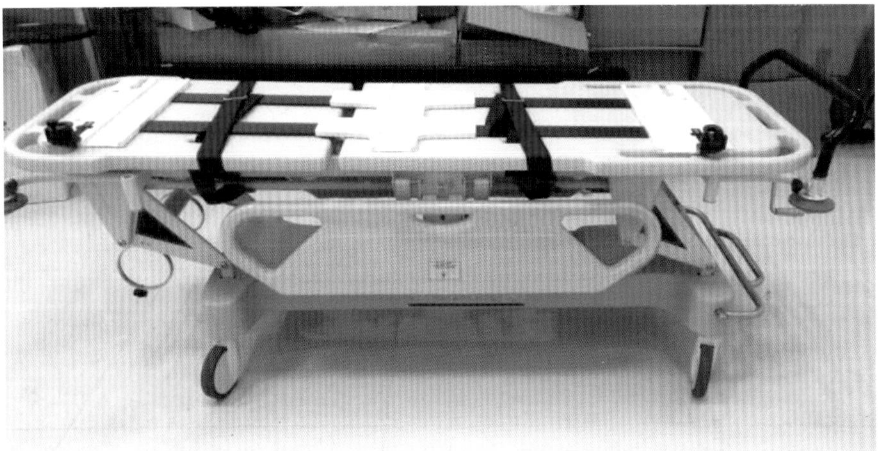

2.转运底板放置于转运模块上并卡好卡扣。

The transfer basic plate is placed on the trolley module and the buckle is stuck.

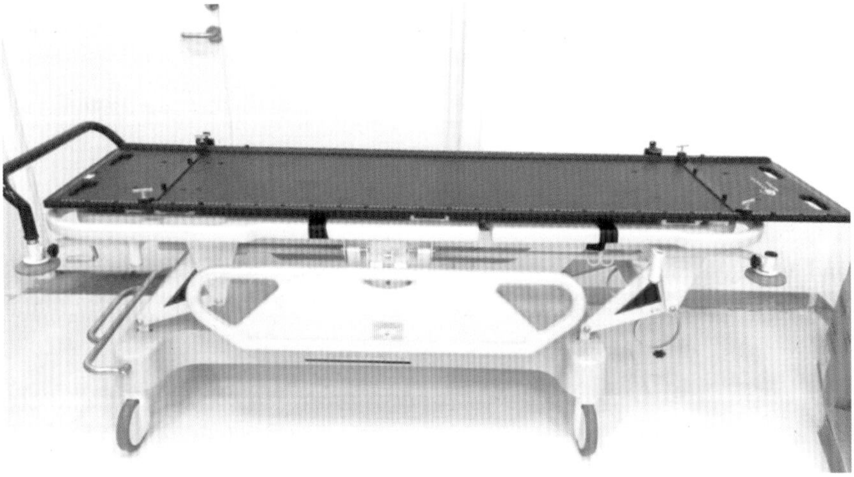

3.将制作好的负压袋卡在转运底板上，患者平躺在负压袋上，扣好体膜。

Place the prepared negative pressure bag on the trolley basic plate and the patient lies on the negative pressure bag, put the body shape on the patient.

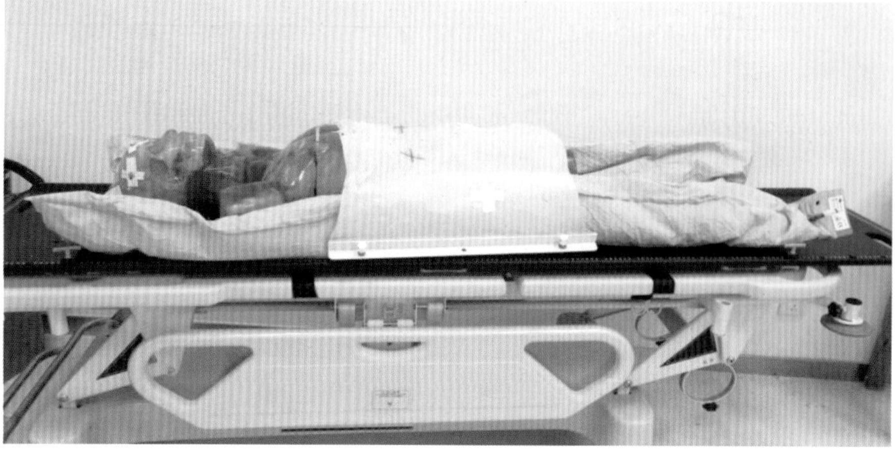

4.松开转运床刹车，将转运车按规定的路线推到治疗室。

Release the trolley brake and push the trolley to the treatment room according to the prescribed route.

5.把lock bar固定在治疗床上，再将另一块转运模块固定在lock bar上，有卡扣的方向靠近90°治疗头。

Fix lock bar on the treatment bed, then fix another piece of transshipment module on the lock bar. A buckle is close to 90 ° in the direction of the nozzle.

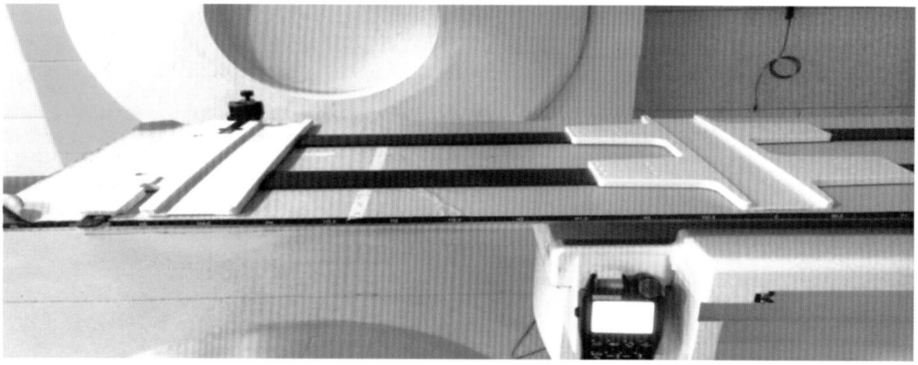

6.将三条滑轨分别置于转运底板的卡槽内。

Place the three slides in the card slot in the trolley basic plate.

7.转运车与治疗床平行且滑轨的另一端卡在治疗床转运模块的卡槽内。

The trolley is in parallel with the treatment bed and the other end of the slide is in the slot of the treatment bed transfer module.

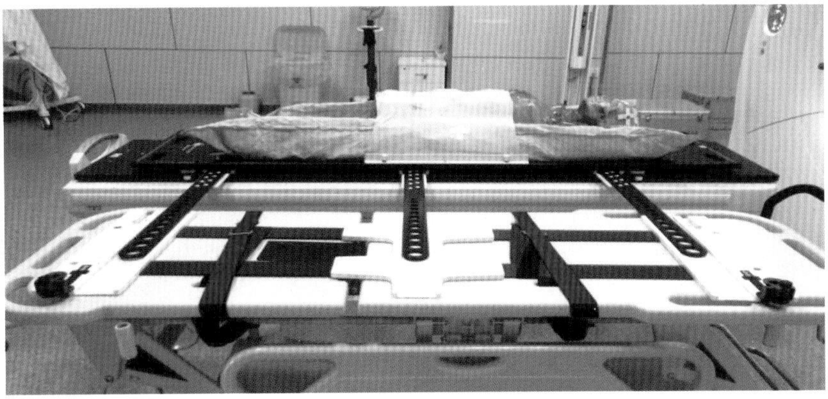

8.松开转运底板的卡扣，缓慢轻推转运底板至治疗床上，卡好卡扣。

Release the buckle of the trolley basic plate and gently push the trolley to the treatment bed, lock the buckle.

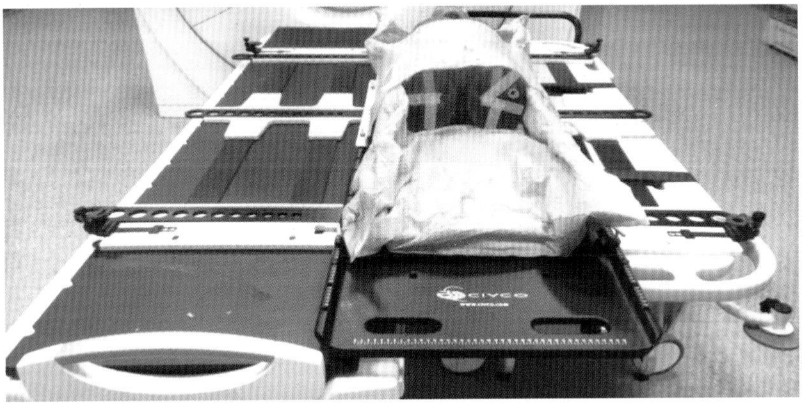

9.升治疗床取下滑轨。

Lift the bed and remove the slide.

10.治疗结束后将滑轨的一端置于治疗床上转运模块的卡槽内，另一端置于转运车转运模块的卡槽内，松开卡扣，缓慢轻推转运底板至转运车上，拧紧卡扣，将患者推出治疗室。

After the treatment, place on side of the slide in the slot of treatment bed transfer module, the other side in the trolley transfer module slot. Loosen the buckle, jog transport floor to the trolley slowly and lightly and then tighten the buckle. We can remove the patient from treatment room.

第18节　碳离子计划（ciPlan）设计标准操作流程

Standard Operating Procedure for Carbon Ion Plan Design

作者：卢小丽　祁英　孟万斌　马霄云

1.在Patient界面，选中患者信息，如图：

Select the patient information in Patient interface, as shown in the figure:

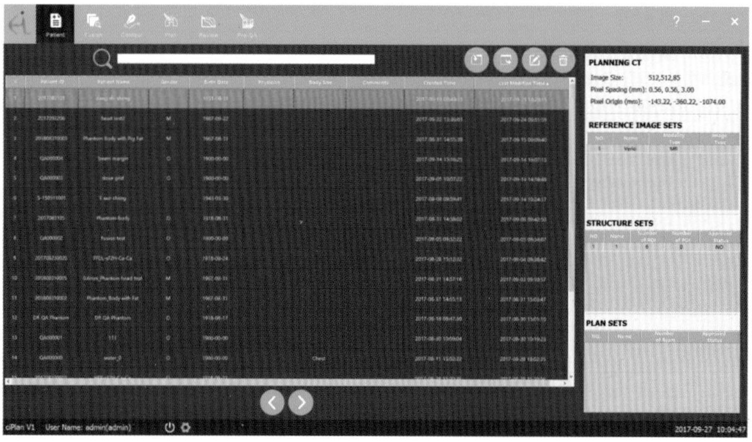

2.点击Contour，进入该界面。如图，在右侧列表框中选择计划CT序列。

Click Contour and enter the interface, as shown in the figure. Select the planned CT sequence in the right list box.

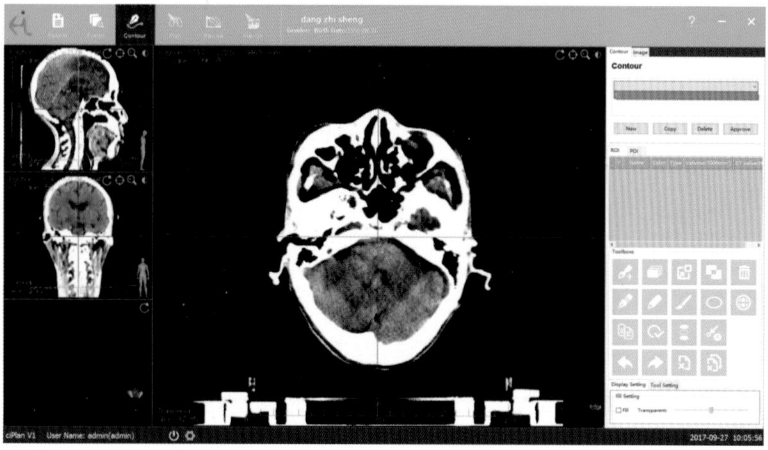

3.点击POI，右侧列表框进入POI界面：

Click POI, and the right list box is changed into the POI interface:

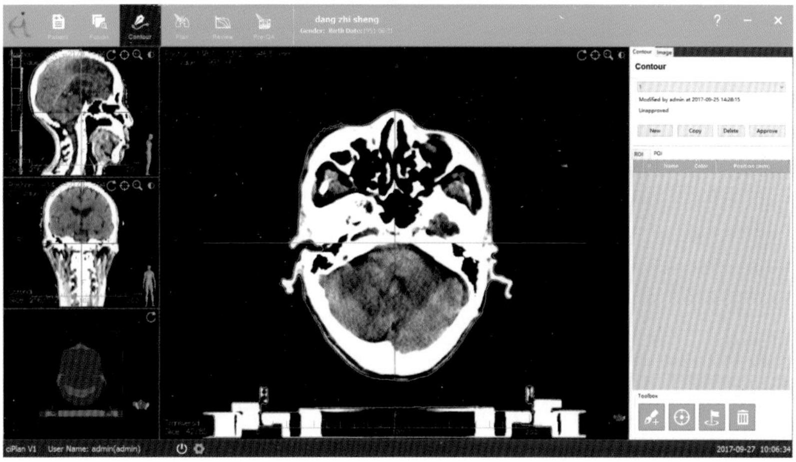

点击，弹出Create POI Dialog窗口，如下图：

Click on , the "Create POI Dialog" window will pop up, as shown in the figure:

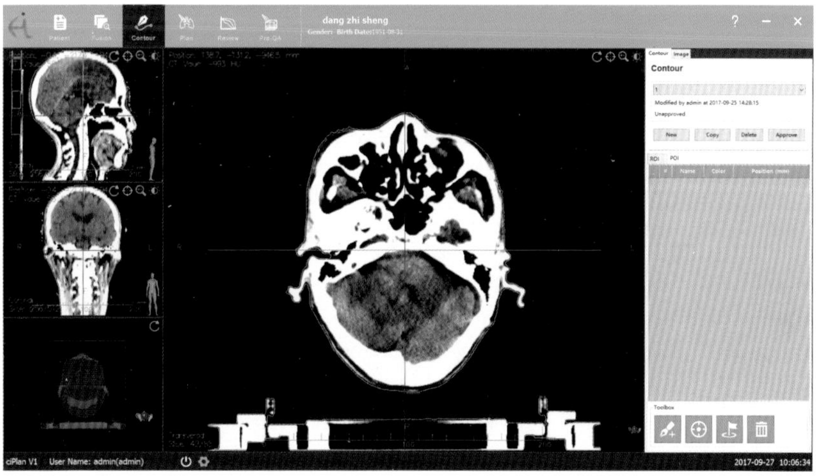

在Name中输入标记点名称，同时可在Manual中手动输入标记点的坐标或点击 通过十字线来确定等中心坐标，如下图。另外，可选择靶区或body的中心为等中心。

Input the name of the marked point in the Name. There are two methods to decide the isocenter coordinate, one is manually inputting the coordinates of the point in Manual, the other is clicking and using cross line to determine the isocenter coordinate, as shown in the figure. In addition, the center of the target or body can be selected as the isocenter.

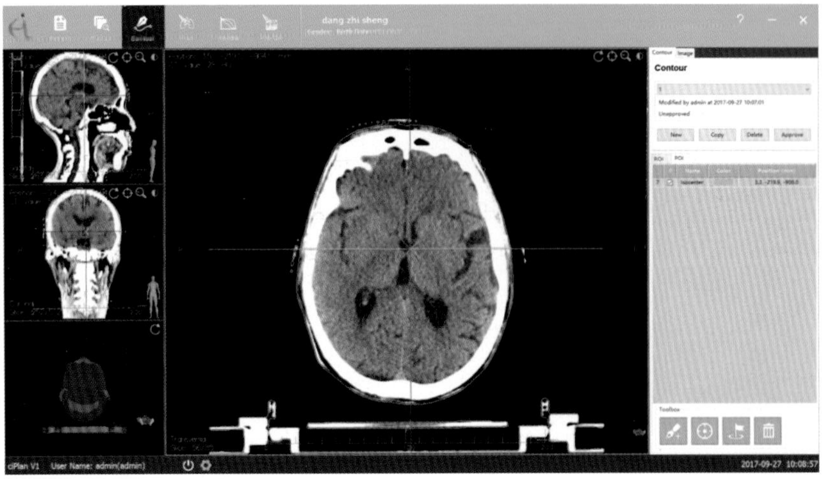

4.进入ROI界面，点击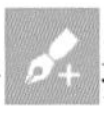打开新建ROI对话框，如图，可直接输入渐渐轮廓名称或从ROI样板中调取轮廓名称。点击进行靶区和正常器官的勾画。

Enter the interface of ROI, Click 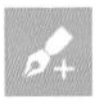 to open the new ROI dialog shown in the figure. There are two ways to add new contour. One is adding one contour directly, the other is selecting the contours from ROI templat. Click 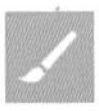 to draw the target area and normal organs.

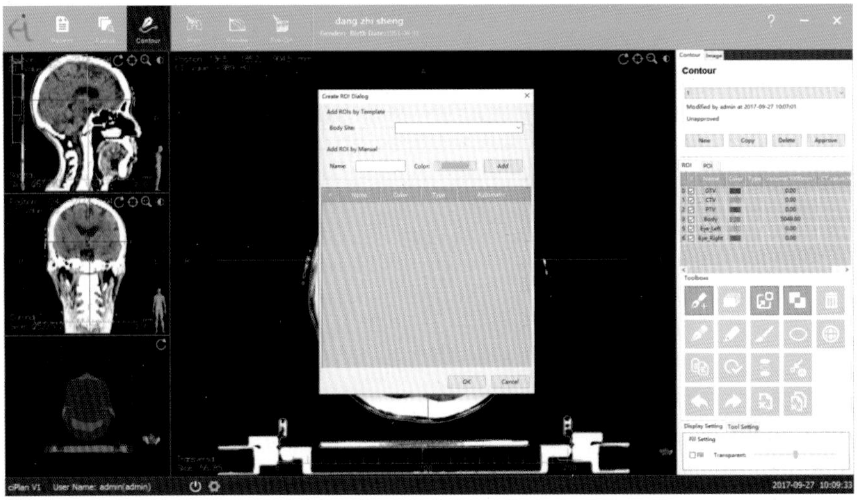

医生对靶区以及正常器官进行勾画和确认。同时给出治疗的处方剂量以及选择合适的治疗方式。确认完成后，点击Approve。

Physicians drew and confirmed the targets and normal tissue. At the same time, the prescription dose and method of the treatment options are given. When the confirmation is complete, click Approve.

5.进入Plan界面，点击New，跳出Crete A New Plan窗口，如下图，在Plan Name中输入计划名称，在Fraction中输入计划次数，在Target & OARS List中选择靶区（一般为最外层的靶区)，点击>>图标，将选择的靶区传入Target Prescription，并在Dose［Gy（RBE）］中输入处方剂量，点击OK。

Enter the Plan interface, click “New” to open the “Crete A New Plan” dialog, as shown in the following figure. Input the plan name in Plan Name and fraction number of the plan in the Fraction, select the target area (the outmost target in general) in Target & OARS List, click the >> symbol to deliver the target area selected to Target Prescription, and input prescription dose in Dose [Gy(RBE)], click OK.

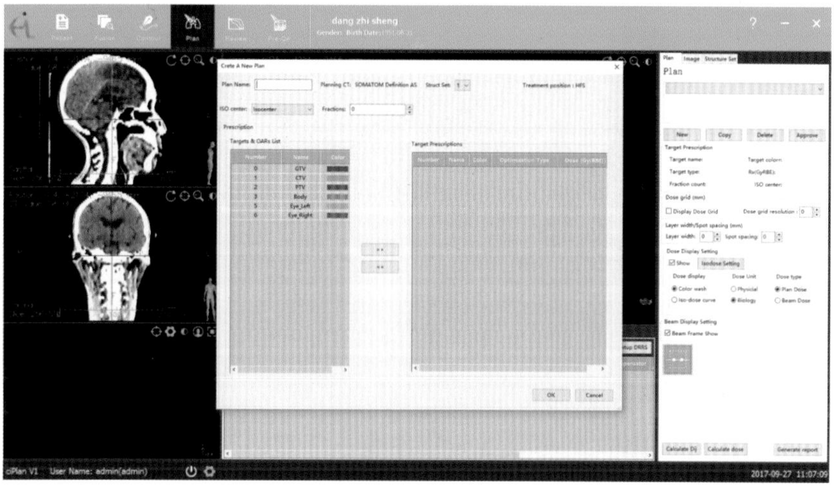

6.点击Add beam，在Add A Beam窗口，在Beam Name中输入射野名称，在Nozzle中选择所需的治疗头，Target中选择相应的治疗靶区，Treatment Type选择治疗方式，选中Compensator选择相应的补偿器（目前只有pmma_40)，Beam Weight一般为[0，1]，Beam Margin一般为[1，6]mm，点击OK，选择合适的床角，点击Compute SOBP，如果有多个野用相同的方法添加射野。点击Calculate dose完成剂量计算，即可显示剂量分布云图。

Click “Add beam”, in the “Add A Beam” dialog, input the name of the beam in Beam Name, and select the suitable nozzle in Nozzle, target area in Target and treatment type in Treatment Type. Select the compensator (only pmma_40 at present) in Compensator, Beam Weight is [0, 1], Beam Margin is [1, 6] mm, and click OK. Input suitable couch angle, and click “Compute SOBP”. If you want to add several fields, the method is the same. Click on “Calculate dose” to finish the dose calculation. The dose-distribution cloud chart is displayed after dose calculation.

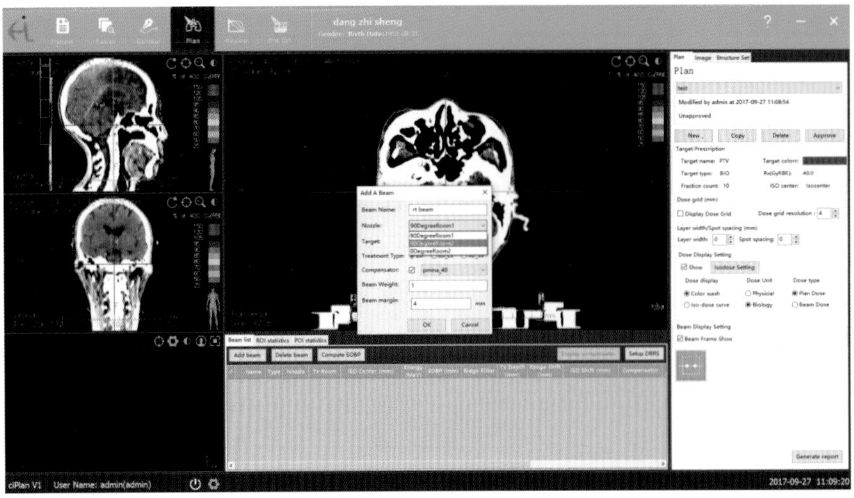

7.在右侧剂量显示设置界面，选择剂量显示方式、剂量类型以及剂量单位。再点击 Isodose setting 设置感兴趣的剂量区域。点击界面左下方视图中的切换按钮，在弹出的列表中选择 DVH，即可在该视图中显示 DVH 图像。点击界面右下方的“Generate Report”生成计划报告。

In the Dose Display Setting interface, we can select the dose display, dose unit and dose type. Click “Isodose setting” to set the interesting dose region. Click the button 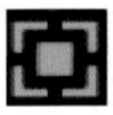 in the lower left view of the interface to select the DVH, and the DVH is displayed. Click “Generate Report” in the lower right of the interface to show the report of the plan。

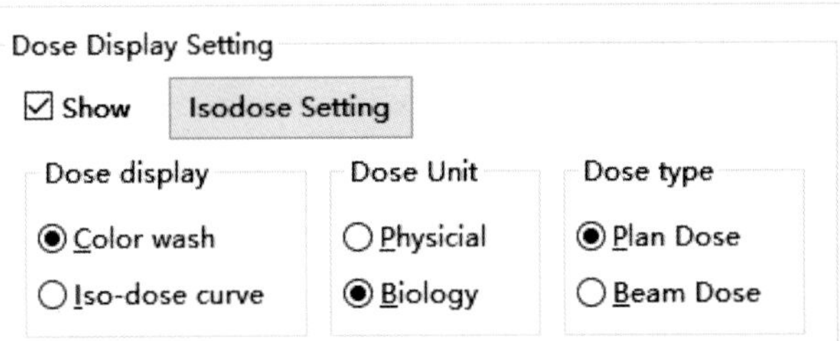

第19节　碳离子放射治疗患者信息导入ciPlan标准操作流程

Standard Operating Procedure for Carbon Ion Radiotherapy Patient Information Importing ciPlan

作者：卢小丽　祁英　孟万斌　马霄云

1.打开ciPlan软件，如下图：

Open ciPlan software, as in the following figure:

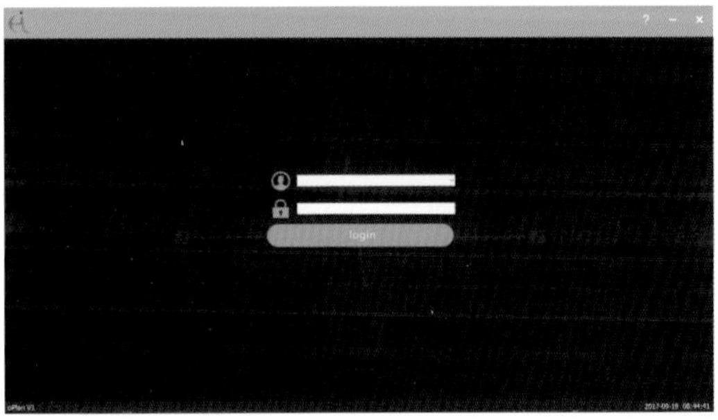

输入用户名：admin，密码：123，点击login登录该系统。

Enter username:admin,Password: 123, click “login” to login the system。

2.进入患者列表界面，如下图：

Enter the patient list interface, as shown in the following figure:

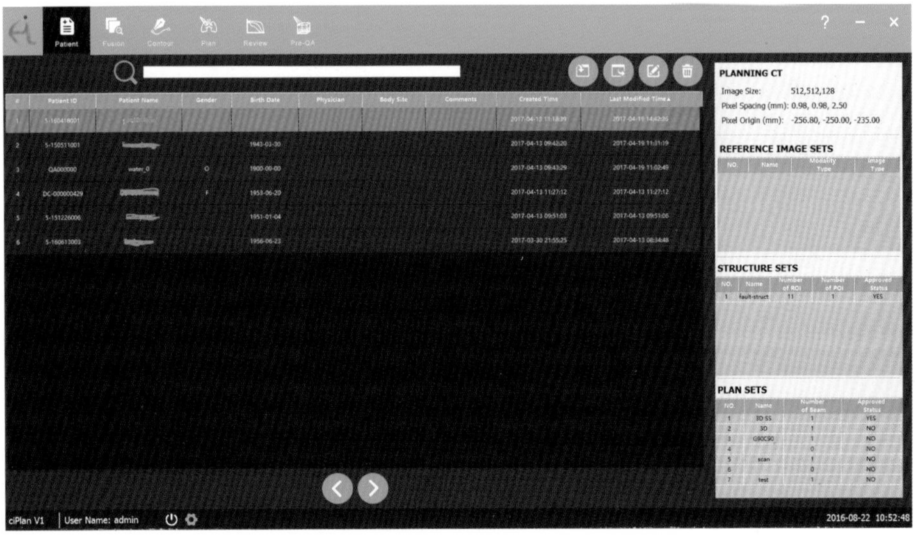

3.点击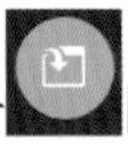图标，会出现如下窗口：

Click , the following window appears.

4.点击Browse，出现如下界面：

Click on “Browse”, so the following interface appears.

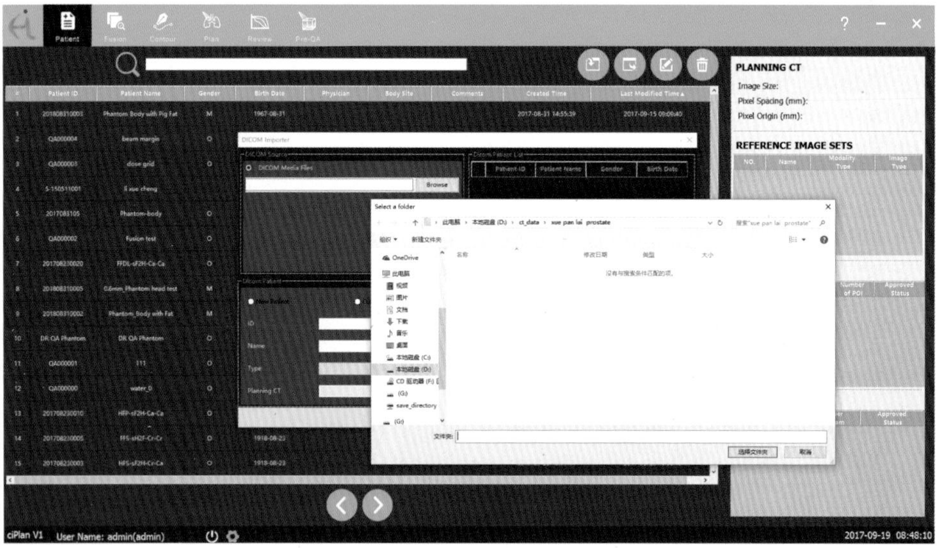

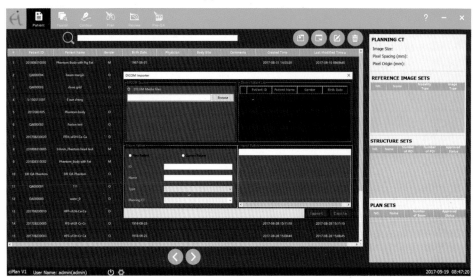

在相应的文件夹中选中需要导入的患者信息。

Select the patient information that needs to be imported in the corresponding folder.

5.选择好信息后，点击窗口右上象限中的患者信息，患者信息显示如下：

After selecting information, click the patient information in the upper right quadrant of the window, and the patient information is shown as below:

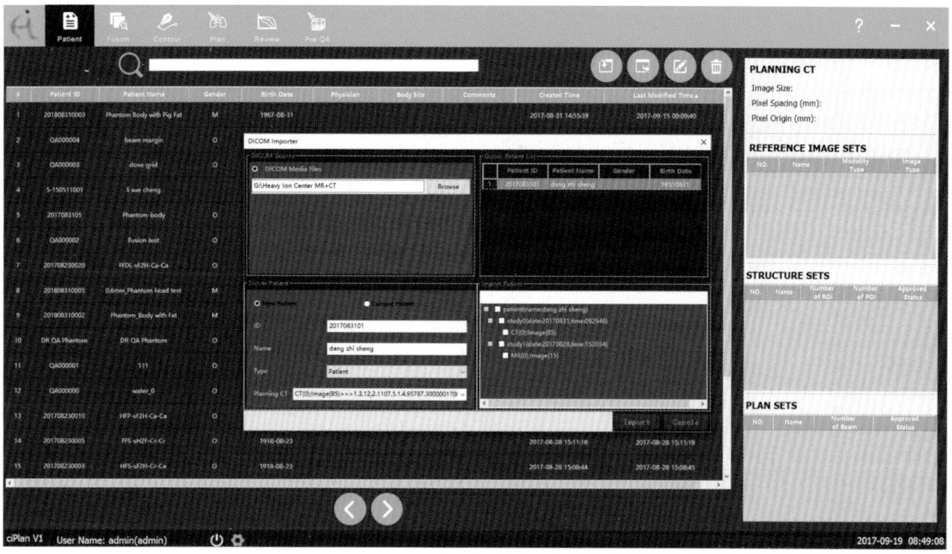

6. 在上图右下象限中勾选上需要导入的CT序列，如下图：

In the lower right quadrant, check the CT sequence that needs to be imported, as shown below:

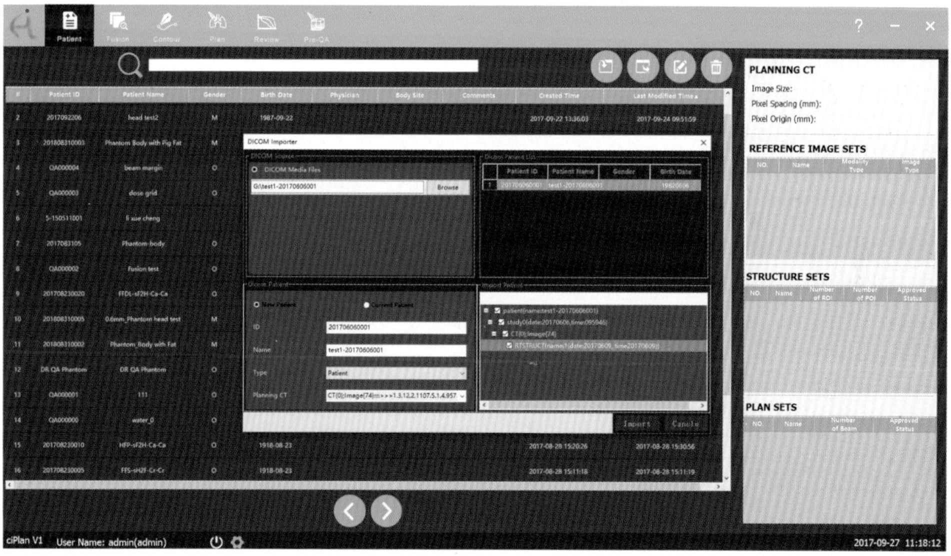

点击Import，至此，患者信息导入完成，在患者信息列表中就可见此患者的ID和名称。

Click "Import", and the import is completed. The patient information including patient ID and name is visible in the list.

第20节 碳离子放射治疗患者信息确认标准操作流程
Standard Operating Procedure for Confirm the Patient's Basic Information for Carbon Ion Radiotherapy

作者：段云龙 祁英 孟万斌 马霄云

治疗执行者必须检查、核对患者首次及疗程中每一次治疗的基本信息，确保患者信息准确无误、完全一致后方可执行治疗。

The therapist must check and confirm the patient's basic information at the first treatment and every treatment in the course, ensure the patient's information is accurate and completely identical. The treatment plan only can be executed at the right situation.

检查核对的项目包括：患者的姓名、性别、年龄、照片、住院号、治疗部位、固定模具、补偿器类型和编号、治疗技术类型、能量档位、治疗总剂量和单次剂量、治疗总次数和剩余次数。如下表所示：

The checking projects including:name, sexuality, age, photo, Admission ID code, treating position, fixing mould, compensator type and code, treating technique type, energy level, total dose and single dose of treating, total fractions and remainder fractions, so on. All the projects are shown in the next table.

患者信息确认表

<table>
<tr><td>姓名</td><td>性别</td><td>年龄</td><td rowspan="4">照片</td></tr>
<tr><td></td><td></td><td></td></tr>
<tr><td>住院号</td><td>治疗部位</td><td>固定模具</td></tr>
<tr><td></td><td></td><td></td></tr>
<tr><td>补偿器类型</td><td>补偿器编号</td><td>治疗技术类型</td><td>能量</td></tr>
<tr><td></td><td></td><td></td><td></td></tr>
<tr><td>疗程总剂量</td><td>单次剂量</td><td>疗程总次数</td><td>剩余次数</td></tr>
<tr><td></td><td></td><td></td><td></td></tr>
</table>

The confirmation form of patient's information

<table>
<tr><td>Name</td><td>Sexuality</td><td>Age</td><td rowspan="4">Photo</td></tr>
<tr><td></td><td></td><td></td></tr>
<tr><td>Admission ID code</td><td>Treating position</td><td>Fixing mould</td></tr>
<tr><td></td><td></td><td></td></tr>
<tr><td>Compensator type</td><td>Compensator ID</td><td>Technique type</td><td>Energy level</td></tr>
<tr><td></td><td></td><td></td><td></td></tr>
<tr><td>Total dose</td><td>Single dose</td><td>Total fractions</td><td>Remainder fractions</td></tr>
<tr><td></td><td></td><td></td><td></td></tr>
</table>

第21节　盆腔、下腹部肿瘤碳离子放射治疗摆位标准操作流程

Standard Operating Procedure for the Position Setting in Carbon Ion Radiotherapy of Pelvic and Lower Abdominal Tumors

作者：段云龙　祁英　孟万斌　马霄云

由于盆腔、下腹部肿瘤的患者治疗部位在身体中段，患者体位固定中一般采用头先进仰卧位、头先进俯卧位、头先进左侧卧位或者头先进右侧卧位。

Because the treatment site of the pelvic cavity, the lower abdomen tumors is in the middle of the body, the head first supine position, head first prone position, head first left side position or head first right position are use in the immobilization of the patient

从便于重复治疗的目标出发，使患者治疗面从正面接近0°或90°的束流方向，从而容易接近治疗机架准直器。

For the goal of repeating the treatment easily, make the patients treating surface from the front close to 0° or 90° beam direction, so as to approach the treatment gantry collimator easily.

选择束流穿射正常组织距离最短的体位，不仅有利于提高放疗的精确性，更有利于减少盆腔、下腹部肠道、双肾、膀胱、股骨头的受照剂量，降低正常组织的副反应。

Select the position when the beam penetrates normal tissue shortestly, and it's beneficial not only to improve the accuracy of radiotherapy, but also to reduce the dose of the pelvic cavity, lower abdomen, double kidney, bladder and femoral head, and reduce the side reaction of normal tissue.

放疗摆位由两名放疗技师操作，具体摆位流程如下：

The radiotherapy position setting is operated by two RT technicians, and the specific positioning procedure is as follows:

（1）告知患者下腹部、盆腔部肿瘤放疗摆位的相关注意事项；

Inform the patients of the position setting of the lower abdomen and pelvic tumors radiotherapy;

（2）根据患者姓名、基本信息、临床诊断的下腹部、盆腔部肿瘤位置，核对使用体位固定板、负压袋和热塑膜上标记的患者信息以及倾斜辅助装置及其所安放的位置，确保与患者本人完全一致；

According to the patient's name and basic information, clinical diagnosis of the lower abdomen, pelvic tumor position, check the patient information of using the position fixing board, the negative pressure bag and the thermoplastic film, and the position of the slanting auxiliary device and the placement, to ensure that the items is in complete agreement with the patient.

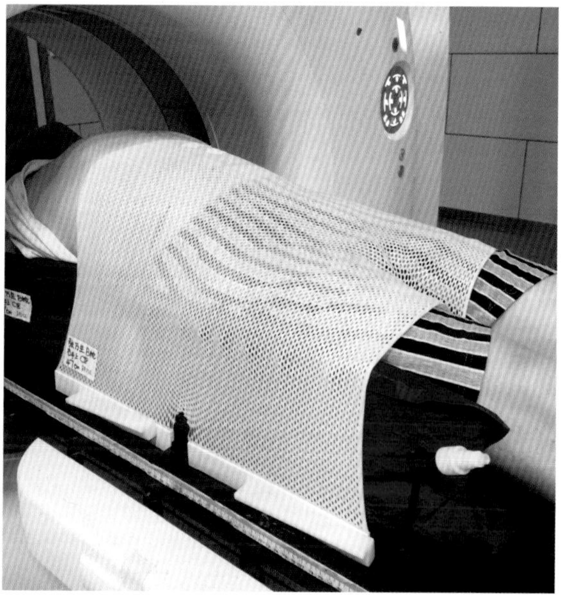

下腹部、盆腔部肿瘤仰卧位治疗体位示意图

The schematic diagram of lower abdomen, pelvic cavity tumor treatment supine position

（3）指导和协助患者躺入体位固定模具，根据体位固定位置及患者最佳自然舒适程度分别采用头先进仰卧位、头先进俯卧位、头先进左侧卧位或者头先进右侧卧位；

Guide and assist the patient lay into the immobilization mold, according to the immobilization location and the patient feeling natural and the most comfortable, head first supine position, head first prone position, head first left side position or head first right side position can be used.

（4）两名放疗技师在治疗床左右两侧，对好体位固定板刻度线、负压袋和患者肢体上的标记线，并适当微调，确保标记线与定位激光灯完全重合；

Both RT technicians are by the left and right sides of the couch, aligning the position fixing board scale line, mark line of negative pressure bag and the patient limbs, and proper fine-tuning, ensure the mark line and positioning laser light coincide.

（5）将热塑膜根据标记位置固定在患者治疗部位，从两侧操作使定位激光线与左侧、右侧和中间的治疗靶线对齐；

The RT technicians fix thermoplastic membrane to the patient's treatment site according to the marked position, and the positioning laser line was aligned with the left, right and middle treatment target line.

（6）使用按钮等固定工具将热塑膜固定在体位固定板上，保持不动，告知患者注意事项并安抚患者，告知患者家属陪员退出机房，关闭防护门，准备实施治疗。

Using the fixed tools such as buttons to fix the thermoplastic film on the position board, keep it still, inform the matters needing attention to the patient and appease him/her, let the family member of the patient exit the machine room, close the guard door for the treatment.

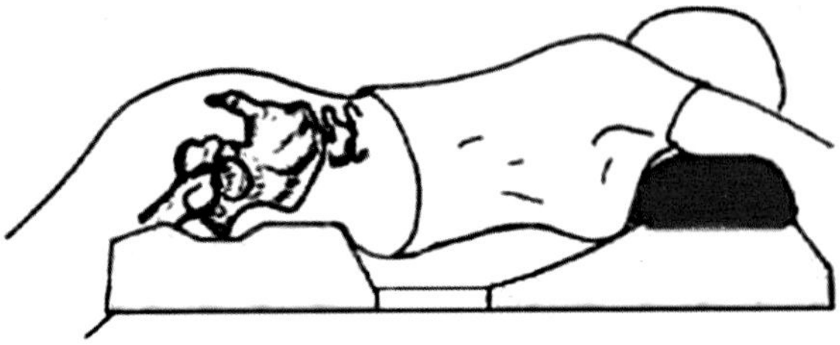

盆腔部肿瘤俯卧位体位治疗固定示意图

The schematic diagram of pelvic tumor prone treatment position

第22节　腿部肿瘤碳离子放射治疗摆位标准操作流程
Standard Operating Procedure for Position Setting in Heavy Ion Radiotherapy of Leg Tumors

作者：段云龙　祁英　孟万斌　马霄云

由于腿部肿瘤的患者身体重量的大部分在躯干，将患者置于脚先进仰卧位、脚先进俯卧位、脚先进左侧卧位或者脚先进右侧卧位。从便于治疗角度出发，使患者治疗面从正面接近0°或90°的束流方向，比较容易接近治疗机架准直器，选择束流穿射正常组织距离最短的体位，不仅有利于提高放疗的精确性，更有利于减少腿部肌肉水肿反应，降低正常组织的副反应。

Because the bulk of the body weight of patients with leg tumors is in the torso, place the patient in foot first supine position, prone position, left side or right side. From the objective of facilitating repeated treatment, make the patients treating surface from the front close to 0° or 90° beam direction, so as to approach the treatment gantry collimator easily. Select the position when the beam penetrates normal tissue shortestly, and it's beneficial not only to improve the accuracy of radiotherapy, but also to reduce the reaction of leg muscle edema and decrease the side reaction of normal tissue.

放疗摆位由两名放疗技师操作，具体摆位流程如下：

The radiotherapy position setting is operated by two RT technicians, and the specific positioning procedure is as follows:

（1）告知患者腿部放疗摆位的相关注意事项；

Inform the patients of the position setting of leg tumor radiotherapy;

（2）根据患者姓名、基本信息、临床诊断的腿部肿瘤位置，核对使用体位固定板、负压袋和热塑膜上标记的患者信息以及倾斜辅助装置及其所安放的位置，确保与患者本人完全一致；

According to the patient's name and basic information, clinical diagnosis of the leg tumor position, check the patient information of using the position fixing board, the negative pressure bag and the thermoplastic film, and the position of the slanting auxiliary device and the placement, to ensure that the items is in complete agreement with the patient.

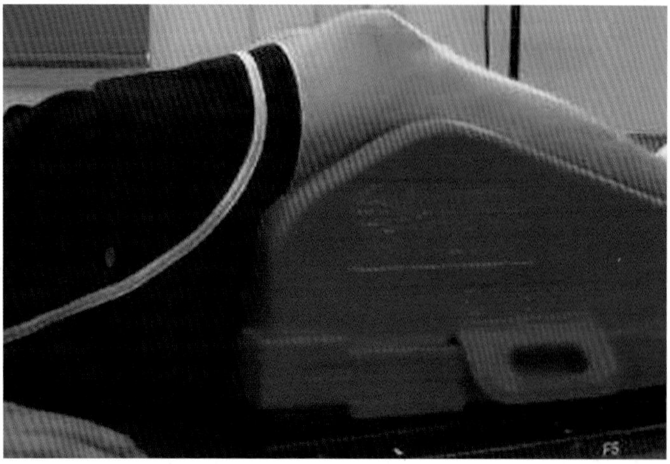

大腿部肿瘤仰卧位治疗体位示意图

The big leg tumor treatment supine position fixed schematic diagram

（3）指导和协助患者躺入体位固定模具，根据体位固定位置及患者最佳自然舒适程度分别选择脚先进仰卧位、脚先进俯卧位、脚先进左侧卧位或者脚先进右侧卧位；

Guide and assist the patient lay into the immobilization mold, according to the immobilization location and the patient feeling natural and the most comfortable, foot first supine position, prone position, left side or right side position are used.

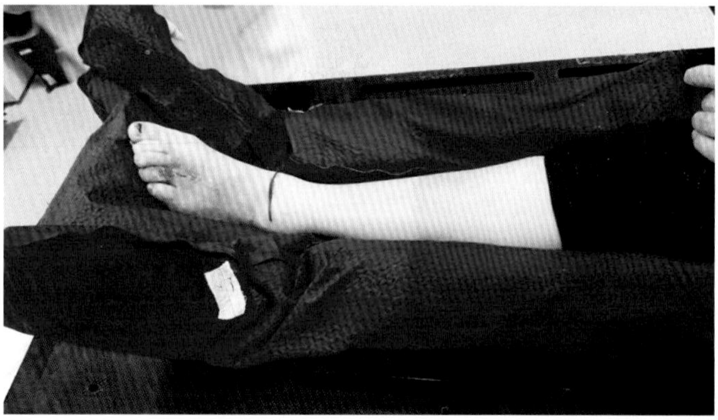

脚部肿瘤仰卧位治疗体位标记示意图

The foot tumor treatment supine position marking schematic diagram

（4）两名放疗技师在治疗床左右两侧，对好体位固定板刻度、负压袋和患者肢体上的标记线，并适当微调，确保标记线与定位激光线完全一致。

Both RT technicians are by the left and right sides of the couch, aligning the position fixing board scale line, mark lin of negative pressure bag and patients limb, and proper fine-tuning, ensure the mark line and positioning laser light coincide.

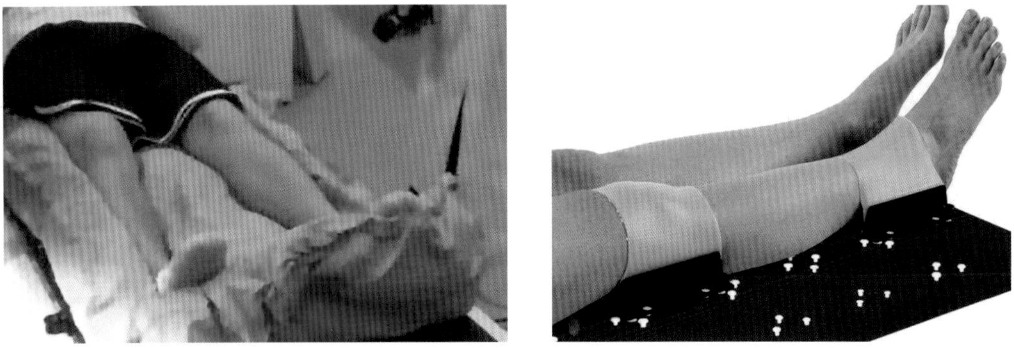

小腿部肿瘤仰卧位治疗体位示意图

The small leg tumor treatment supine position schematic diagram

（5）将热塑膜根据标记位置固定在患者治疗部位，从两侧操作，使定位激光线与左侧、右侧和中间的治疗靶线对齐；

The RT technicians fix thermoplastic membrane to the patient's treatment site according to the marked position, and the positioning laser line was aligned with the left, right and middle treatment target line.

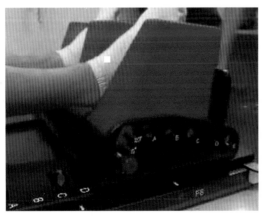

脚部肿瘤仰卧位治疗体位示意图

The foot tumor supine treatment position schematic diagram

（6）使用按钮等固定附件将热塑膜固定在体位固定板上，保持不动，告知患者注意事项并安抚患者，告知患者家属陪员退出机房，关闭防护门，准备实施治疗。

Using the fixed tools such as buttons to fix the thermoplastic film on the position board, keep it still, inform the matters needing attention to the patient and appease him/her, let the family member of the patient exit the machine room, close the guard door for the treatment.

第23节　手部肿瘤碳离子放射治疗摆位标准操作流程

Standard Operating Procedure for the Position Setting in Carbon Ion Beam Radiotherapy of Arm Tumors

作者：段云龙　祁英　孟万斌　马霄云

手部肿瘤采用碳离子放疗，将患者手臂伸展，置于头先进仰卧位、头先进俯卧位、头先进左侧卧位或者头先进右侧卧位，或站立在治疗床前端把患侧的手放置于体位固定板上。

As for the arm tumor carbon ion radiotherapy, put the patient's arm outstretched, in head first supine, prone, right side, left side bits, or let the patient stand in front side of the treatment bed whose hands are placed on the fixed board.

从便于治疗角度出发，使患者治疗面从正面接近0°或90°的束流方向，比较容易接近治疗机架准直器，选择束流穿射正常组织距离最短的体位，不仅有利于提高放疗的精确性，更有利于减少肌肉组织的受照剂量降低正常组织的副反应。

For the goal of repeating the treatment easily, make the patients treating surface from the front close to 0 ° or 90 ° beam direction, so as to approach the treatment gantry collimator easily. Select the position when the beam penetrates normal tissue shortestly, and it is beneficial not only to improve the accuracy of radiotherapy, but also to reduce the reaction of arm muscle edema and decrease the side reaction of normal tissue.

放疗摆位由两名放疗技师操作，具体摆位流程如下：

The radiotherapy position setting is operated by two RT technicians, and the specific positioning procedure is as follows:

（1）告知患者手部肿瘤放疗摆位的相关注意事项；

Inform the patients of position setting of the hand tumor radiotherapy.

（2）根据患者姓名、基本信息、临床诊断的手部肿瘤位置，核对使用体位固定板、负压袋和热塑膜上标记的患者信息以及倾斜辅助装置及其所安放的位置，确保与患者本人完全一致；

According to the patient's name and basic information, clinical diagnosis of the leg tumor position, check the patient information of using the position fixing board, the negative pressure bag and the thermoplastic film, and the position of the slanting auxiliary device and the placement, to ensure that the items are in complete agreement with the patient.

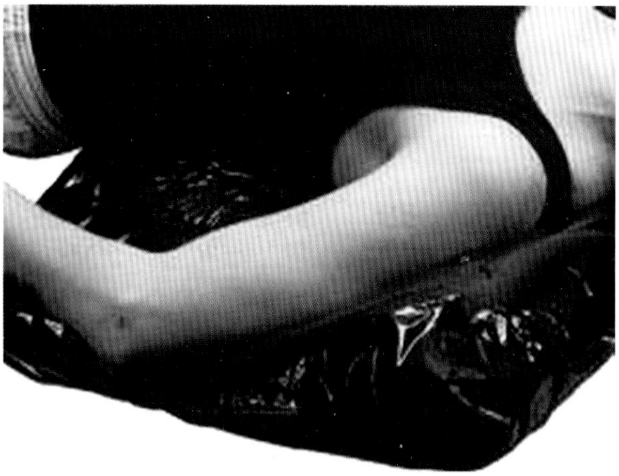

手部肿瘤仰卧位治疗体位示意图

The hand tumor treatment supine position schematic diagram

（3）指导和协助患者进入体位固定模具，根据体位固定位置患者最佳自然舒适程度分别选择头先进仰卧位、头先进俯卧位、头先进左侧卧位、头先进右侧卧位；或者患者站立在治疗床前端，将左手臂或右手臂放置在体位固定板、负压袋上，根据防护需要指导患者戴铅帽、穿铅衣、铅围脖、围裙或使用铅橡胶等防护设备覆盖、遮挡非照射的重要器官部位；

Guide and assist the patient to get into the position fixed mold, according to the fixed position location and the patient feeling natural and the most comfortable, head first supine position, head first prone position, head first left side or head first right side position can be used. Or let the patient stand at the front of the couch, placing the left arm on right arm on the position plate, the negative pressure bag and the protection requires to instruct the patient to wear a lead hat, lead suit, lead neck, an apron, or use of lead rubber to cover the vital organs of the non-irradiated parts.

（4）两名放疗技师在治疗床左右两侧，对好体位固定板刻度、负压袋和患者手臂上的标记线，并适当微调，确保标记线与定位激光线完全一致；

Both RT technicians are by left and right sides of the couch, aligning the position fixing board scale line, mark line of negative pressure bag and of the patients with limb, and proper fine-tuning, ensure the mark line and positioning laser light coincide.

（5）将热塑膜根据标记位置固定在患者治疗部位，从两侧操作使定位激光线与左侧、右侧和中间的治疗靶线对齐；

The RT technicians fix thermoplastic membrane to the patient's treatment site according to the marked position, and the positioning laser line was aligned with the left, right and middle treatment target line.

（6）使用按钮等固定工具将热塑膜固定在体位固定板上，保持不动，告知患者注意事项并安抚患者，告知患者家属陪员退出机房，关闭防护门，准备实施治疗。

Using the fixed tools such as buttons to fix the thermoplastic film on the position board, keep it still, inform the matters needing attention to the patient and appease him/her, let the family member of the patient exit the machine room, close the guard door for the treatment.

第24节　其他部位肿瘤碳离子放射治疗摆位标准操作流程
Standard Operating Procedure for Position Setting in Carbon Ion Radiotherapy of Other Parts Tumors

作者：段云龙　祁英　孟万斌　马霄云

根据其他部位肿瘤的治疗位置，从便于重复治疗的目标出发，使患者治疗面从正面接近0°或90°的束流方向，容易接近治疗机架准直器，选择束流穿射正常组织距离最短的体位，不仅有利于提高放疗的精确性，更有利于减少其他部位危及器官的受照剂量，降低正常组织的副反应。

Depending on the location of the tumor in other sites, for the goal of repeating treatment easily, make the patients treating surface from the front close to 0 ° or 90 ° beam direction, so as to approach the treatment gantry collimator easily, selecting the position when the beam penetrates normal tissue shortestly, and it's beneficial not only to improve the accuracy of radiotherapy, but also to reduce the reaction of normal tissue.

放疗摆位由两名放疗技师操作，具体摆位流程如下：

The radiotherapy position setting is operated by two RT technicians, and the specific positioning procedure is as follows:

（1）告知患者其他部位放疗摆位的相关注意事项；

Inform the patients of the position setting of radiotherapy of tumor in other site;

（2）根据患者姓名、基本信息、临床诊断的其他部位肿瘤位置，核对使用体位固定板、负压袋、热塑膜上标记的患者信息以及倾斜辅助装置及其所安放的位置，确保与患者本人完全一致；

According to the patient's name and basic information, clinical diagnosis of the other tumor position, check the patient information of using the position fixing board, the negative pressure bag and the thermoplastic film, and the position of the slanting auxiliary device and the placement, to ensure that the items are in complete agreement with the patient.

（3）指导和协助患者进入体位固定模具，根据体位固定位置及患者最佳自然舒适程度分别采用相对应的固定体位；

Guide and assist the patient to get into the position fixed mold, according to the fixed position location and the patient feeling natural and the most comfortable, the best positioning is used.

（4）两名放疗技师在治疗床左右两侧，对好体位固定板刻度线、负压袋和患者肢体上的标记线，并适当微调，确保标记线与定位激光灯完全重合；

Both RT technicians are by the left and right sides of the couch，aligning the position fixing board scale line, mark line negative pressure bag and mark line in the patients with limb，and proper fine-tuning，ensure the mark line and positioning laser light coincide.

（5）将热塑膜根据标记位置固定在患者治疗部位，从两侧操作，使定位激光线与左侧、右侧和中间的治疗靶线对齐；

The RT technicians fix thermoplastic membrane to the patient's treatment site according to the marked position，and the positioning laser line was aligned with the left，right and middle treatment target line.

（6）使用按钮等固定工具将热塑膜固定在体位固定板上，保持不动，告知患者注意事项并安抚患者，告知患者家属陪员退出机房，关闭防护门，准备实施治疗。

Using the fixed tools such as buttons to fix the thermoplastic film on the position board，keep it still，inform the matters needing attention to the patient and appease him/her，let the family member of the patient exit the machine room，close the guard door for the treatment.

第25节　碳离子放射治疗患者转运出治疗室及下床标准操作流程

Standard Operating Procedure for Patients Transfering from the Treatment Room and Getting off Bed in Carbon Ion Rodiotherapy

作者：王开平　祁英　孟万斌　马霄云

1.治疗结束后把转运车推至治疗床旁，将滑轨的一端置于治疗床上转运模块的卡槽内，另一端置于转运床转运模块的卡槽内，松开卡扣缓慢轻推转运底板至转运床上，拧紧卡扣。

Push the transport vehicles to treatment bet after treatment, put one end of the slide rail on transport module card slot treatment bed, the other side on transport bed module card slot, loosen the card buckle, jog transshipment base plate to transshipment on the bed slowly, tighten the clasp.

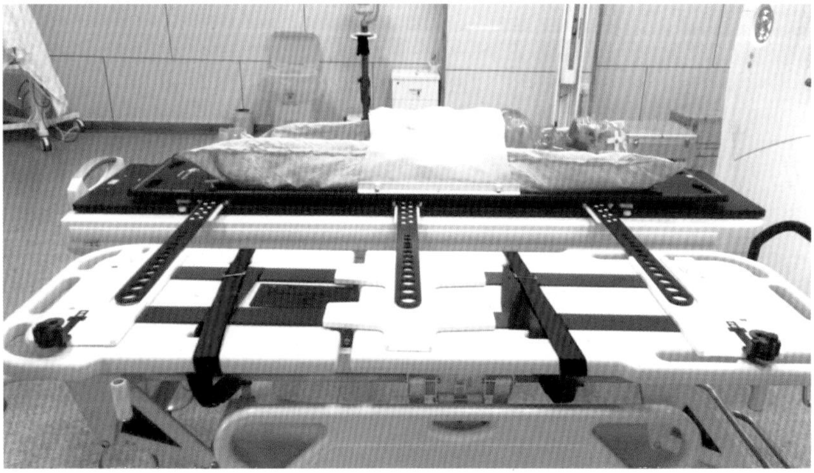

2.将患者推出治疗室到更衣室。

Push the patient from the treatment room to the preparation room.

3.取除体膜及辅助装置。

Remove thermoplastic and auxiliary devices.

4.将患者从负压袋内扶起并搀扶下床。

Lift the patient from the gray bag and assist him to get off the bed.

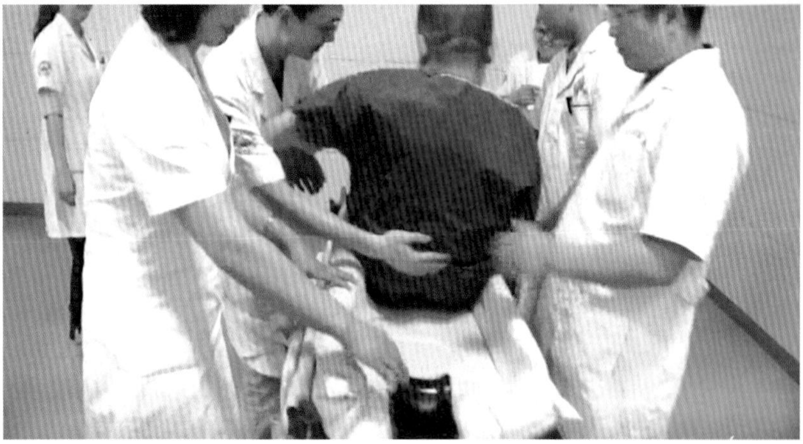

5.协助病人穿好衣服，讲清注意事项及治疗时间。

Help the patient to wear clothes and inform him of notes and time of treatment.

6.送病人走出更衣间。

Help the patient to walk out of preparation room.

第26节　碳离子放射治疗四肢肿瘤及其他部位肿瘤体位固定标准操作流程

Standard Operating Procedure for Immobilization in Carbon Ion Radiotherapy of Limbs and Other Parts Tumors

作者：王开平　祁英　孟万斌　马霄云

下肢肿瘤患者的体位固定大致可分为两步：即真空负压袋塑型和热塑膜塑型。

The immobilization of lower limb tumor patients can be divided into two steps: vacuum bag shaping and thermoplastic mask shaping.

1　真空负压袋塑型

(Vacuum bag shaping)

真空负压袋内部由小的聚苯乙烯珠填充，真空袋垫在患者需要固定的下肢形成一个坚硬的、舒适的襁褓，以起到固定病人的作用。

The vacuum bag is filled with small polystyrene beads and the vacuum bag is designed to form a solid, comfortable swaddling in the patient's lower extremities to help stabilize the patient.

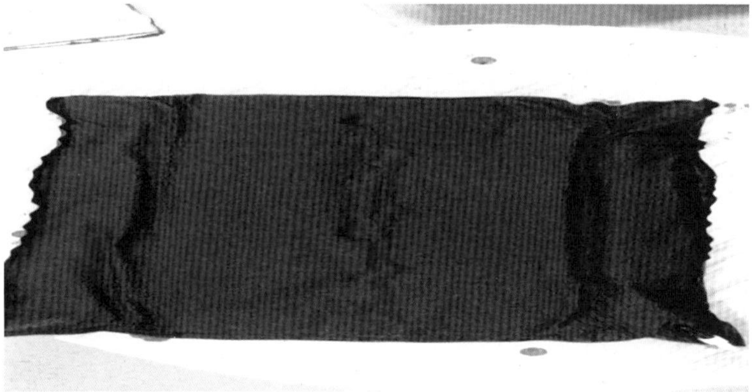

真空负压袋的制作技术要求和传统的光子放疗真空负压袋的制作技术要求基本相同，可根据光子的经验去完成真空负压袋的制作。

The production technology demand of vacuum bag is the same as that of the traditional photon radiotherapy and the bag can be made according to the experience of photon radiotherapy.

2 患者定位

(Patient Positioning)

病人预约定位时间后，按医生要求准备好真空负压袋，让已经更换好病员服的患者脱掉拖鞋，将需要固定的患侧下肢放在真空负压袋上，调整病人的体位以病人最舒适、保持时间最长的姿势为最佳。

After appointment, according to the requirements of the doctor, prepare vacuum bag, let the prepared patient take off his shoes and socks, wear special clothing and put the diseased side on the vacuum bag. Adjust the position of the patient which makes the patient feel most comfortable, and can keep the longest time.

（1）置患者于负压袋最正中，卷起负压袋的边缘部分，紧贴于患侧下肢两侧。

Put the patient in the middle of the vacuum bag. Roll up the edge of the vacuum bag and cling to the side of the lower extremities.

（2）真空负压袋初步塑型后，打开气泵，连接阀门，进行抽真空。这个阶段是最为关键的阶段，操作人员要仔细观察真空袋的硬化过程，确保真空袋每个部位的硬化都是我们预设的形状。

After the vacuum bag is initially molded, turn on air pump, connect valve and vacuum. This stage is the most critical stage. The operators should carefully observe the hardening process of the vacuum bag to ensure that the hardening of each part of the vacuum bag is the shape we preset.

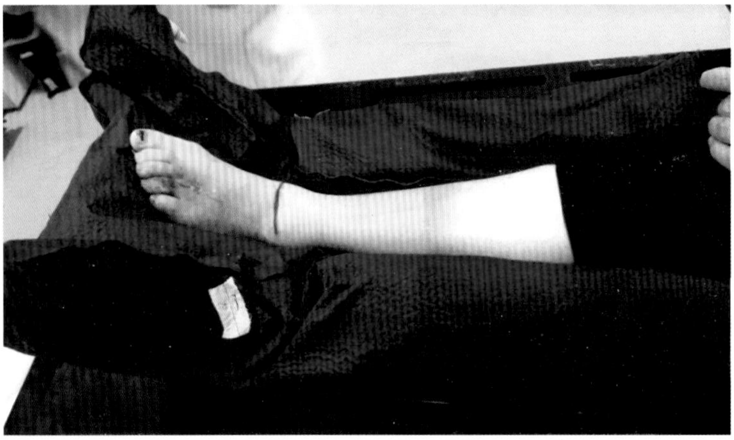

（3）确保真空袋的制作准确无误地完成并记录真空压力，关闭气泵。

Make sure the vacuum bag is finished correctly and record the vacuum pressure and shut off the air pump.

（4）制作完成后记录该患者真空负压袋的全部信息。真空负压袋有自己配套使用的便捷标签，切记详细记录患者信息，如：左右患侧肢，真空袋气压等等。

After the vacuum bag is finished, the whole information of vacuum bag must be recorded. There is a special label for the vacuum bag. Remember to record the information of the patient in detail, such as the left and right side of the limb, the vacuum bag pressure, etc.

3 固定模具操作流程

(Manufacturing process of immobilization)

（1）将准备好的热塑膜放入恒温水箱（70 ℃）中加热，使其由硬变软可以随意拉伸。

Heat the mask in the thermostat (70°C) to make it soft and easy to stretch.

（2）将烫好的热塑膜根据病人病灶的位置固定在患者下肢上。

Fix the softened thermoplastic mask to the lower limb of the patient.

（3）等待10～15分钟至体膜收缩变凉变硬无自然形变时，标记好病人信息及初始定位标记点。

Wait for 10 to 15 minutes until the thermoplastic mask shrinks and becomes cool and hard without the natural deformation. Mark the patient information and the initial positioning mark.

（4）确认信息无误后将膜具取下，放置在固定位置。

After confirming the information, remove the mask and place it in a dedicated position.

第27节 碳离子放射治疗计划命名标准操作流程
Standard Operating Procedure for Carbon Ion Radiotherapy Plan Naming

作者：马霄云 祁英 孟万斌 马霄云

为规范碳离子放射治疗计划的名称，使所有工作人员能一目了然地了解该物理计划的基本情况，特制定本命名规则。本规则适用于高能碳离子放射治疗计划系统（ci_Plan）。

In order to regulate the naming procedure of the carbon ion radiotherapy treatment plan, so that every staff can understand the basic information of this plan clearly, hereby we make this naming procedure. This procedure is suitable for high energy carbon ion radiotherapy planning system, which is named as "ci_Plan".

治疗计划的命名格式为：

The naming format of the treatment plan is :

PlanN_AA_BM_PO_DATE

如：一例单野头部计划可命名为：Plan1_2D_1B_Head_20171101

一例两野腹部计划可命名为：Plan2_2DLS_2B_Abdo_20171218

For example:

One single beam head treatment plan can be named as : Plan1_2D_1B_Head_20171101

One two beams abdomen treatment plan can be named as:

Plan2_2DLS_2B_Abdo_20171218

以下为详细命名规则：

The detailed naming protocol is as following:

① N：1、2、3……为计划的序号，如第一个计划为Plan1_...，第二个为Plan_2...，以此类推。

N：1、2、3... is the series number of the plan, for example: the first plan is Plan1_..., The second one is Plan_2..., and so on.

② AA：束流扫描方式，有三种：2D，2DLS，3DSS，如：Plan1_2D_...，Plan2_2DLS_...，Plan3_3DSS_...

AA：the beam scanning mode, there are three ways: 2D，2DLS，3DSS，For example:

Plan1_2D_...，Plan2_2DLS_...，Plan3_3DSS_...

③ BM：射野数目，如有一个野，则为1B，有两个野，为2B，如：Plan1_2D_1B_...，Plan2_2DLS_2B_...，以此类推。

BM：the beam number, if there is only one beam, it will be 1B. If there are two beams, it will be 2B. For example: Plan1_2D_1B_...，Plan2_2DLS_2B_...， and so on.

④ PO：患者大体的照射部位，如头部为Head，胸部为Chest，腹部为Abdo，盆腔为Pelvis等，如Plan1_2D_1B_Head_...， Plan2_2DLS_2B_Abdo_...，以此类推。

PO：the approximate position of the irradiation. For example, a head patient, the PO will be “Head”, a chest patient will be “Chest”, an abdomen patient will be “Abdo”, a pelvic patient will be “Pelvis”, etc. So the plan will be named as Plan1_2D_1B_Head_..., Plan2_2DLS_2B_Abdo_...， and so on.

⑤ DATE：制作计划的日期，如Plan1_2D_1B_Head_20171101， Plan2_2DLS_2B_Abdo_20171218.

DATE： the date of making this treatment plan, for example: Plan1_2D_1B_Head_20171101， Plan2_2DLS_2B_Abdo_20171218. etc.

附：

1.碳离子放射治疗计划申请单模板

<table>
<tr><td colspan="6">碳离子放射治疗计划申请单
甘肃重离子医院</td></tr>
<tr><td>患者姓名：</td><td></td><td>性别：</td><td></td><td>年龄：</td><td></td></tr>
<tr><td>主管医生：</td><td></td><td>病区：</td><td colspan="3"></td></tr>
<tr><td>诊断：</td><td colspan="5"></td></tr>
<tr><td>分期：</td><td></td><td>其他：</td><td colspan="3"></td></tr>
<tr><td colspan="6">之前是否接受过X射线、质子、重离子等放射治疗？（请勾选）是　否</td></tr>
<tr><td>如之前接受过放射治疗，请描述具体情况：</td><td colspan="5"></td></tr>
<tr><td colspan="6">本次碳离子放射治疗剂量处方</td></tr>
<tr><td>治疗方式（请勾选）：</td><td colspan="5">2D　2DLS　3DSS</td></tr>
<tr><td>患者体位固定方式：</td><td colspan="5"></td></tr>
<tr><td rowspan="2">靶区剂量：
Gy（RBE）</td><td colspan="3"></td><td colspan="2">Gy（RBE）</td></tr>
<tr><td colspan="3"></td><td colspan="2">Gy（RBE）</td></tr>
<tr><td rowspan="7">OAR限量：
Gy（RBE）</td><td colspan="5"></td></tr>
<tr><td colspan="5"></td></tr>
<tr><td colspan="5"></td></tr>
<tr><td colspan="5"></td></tr>
<tr><td colspan="5"></td></tr>
<tr><td colspan="5"></td></tr>
<tr><td colspan="5"></td></tr>
<tr><td>特殊要求：</td><td colspan="5"></td></tr>
<tr><td>靶区勾画签名：</td><td colspan="5">年　月　日</td></tr>
<tr><td>靶区确认签名：</td><td colspan="5">年　月　日</td></tr>
<tr><td>计划设计签名：</td><td colspan="5">年　月　日</td></tr>
<tr><td>计划审核签名：</td><td colspan="5">年　月　日</td></tr>
</table>

2.物理师放射治疗计划确认单模板。

<table>
<tr><td colspan="6">物理师放射治疗计划确认单
甘肃重离子医院</td></tr>
<tr><td>患者姓名：</td><td>Zhang San</td><td>性别：</td><td>男</td><td>年龄：</td><td>77</td></tr>
<tr><td>Patient ID：</td><td>2017083001</td><td colspan="2">Beam Type:</td><td colspan="2">2D</td></tr>
<tr><td>Treatment plan name：</td><td colspan="5">Plan1_2D_1B_20170831</td></tr>
<tr><td>Contour name:</td><td>CT_7</td><td colspan="2">Target name:</td><td colspan="2">PTV</td></tr>
<tr><td>Rx (Gy RBE):</td><td>50</td><td colspan="2">Fractions:</td><td colspan="2">10</td></tr>
<tr><td>Number of beams:</td><td>1</td><td colspan="2">Treatment room:</td><td colspan="2">Room 1</td></tr>
<tr><td colspan="6">
<table>
<tr><td></td><td>Beam 1</td><td>Beam 2</td><td>Beam 3</td></tr>
<tr><td>Nozzle name:</td><td>90 Degree Room1</td><td></td><td></td></tr>
<tr><td>Nozzle angle:</td><td>90 degree</td><td></td><td></td></tr>
<tr><td>Couch angle:</td><td>0 degree</td><td></td><td></td></tr>
<tr><td>MLC angle:</td><td>0 degree</td><td></td><td></td></tr>
<tr><td>Energy:</td><td>120.0 MeV</td><td></td><td></td></tr>
<tr><td>Ridge filter:</td><td>RF60</td><td></td><td></td></tr>
<tr><td>Compensator name:</td><td>PMMA40</td><td></td><td></td></tr>
<tr><td>Range shifter:</td><td>30 mm</td><td></td><td></td></tr>
</table>
</td></tr>
<tr><td>Plan approved:</td><td>yes</td><td colspan="2">Designed by:</td><td colspan="2">Ma Xiaoyun</td></tr>
<tr><td>Checked by:</td><td>Meng Wanbin</td><td colspan="2">Date:</td><td colspan="2">2017年8月31</td></tr>
</table>

第28节　高压注射器标准操作流程
Standard Operating Procedure for High Pressure Syringe

作者：陈喆　李菊琴　祁英　孟万斌　马霄云

本注射器系统适用于在静脉侧低压下注射X射线碘造影剂，然后跟进盐水的程序，和CT扫描仪联合使用。有关特定的扫描仪和其他相关设备的使用说明，请您参照随那些设备一同提供的手册。

This injector system is suitable for use in low pressure against the side of intravenous injection of X - ray iodine contrast agent, and then follow up brine process, and used in combination with CT scanners. As for specific instructions on the use of the scanner and other related equipment, please refer to the manual that provided with equipment.

1.打开电源开关。

Turn on the power switch.

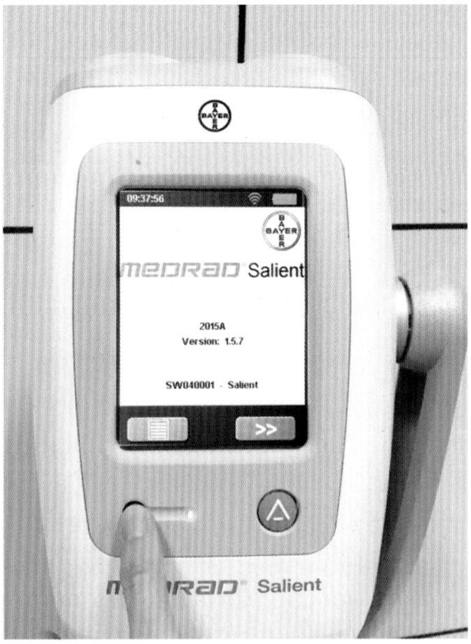

2.安装针筒，抽取造影剂、生理盐水。

Install the syringe，extract contrast agent and saline.

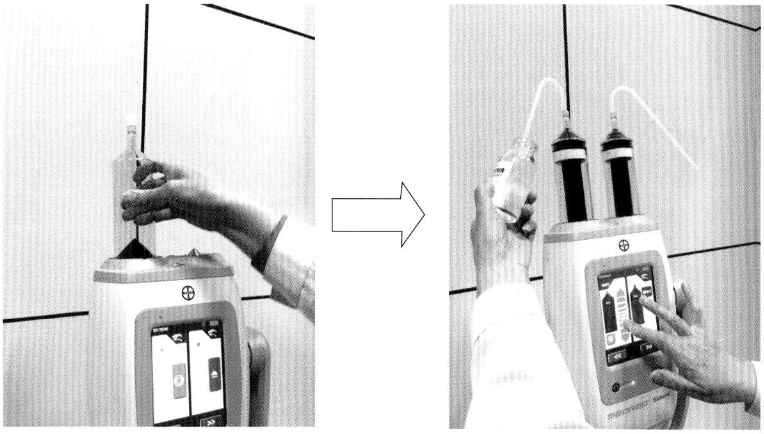

3.接高压连接线，排空气体。

Connect the high voltage connection line and empty air.

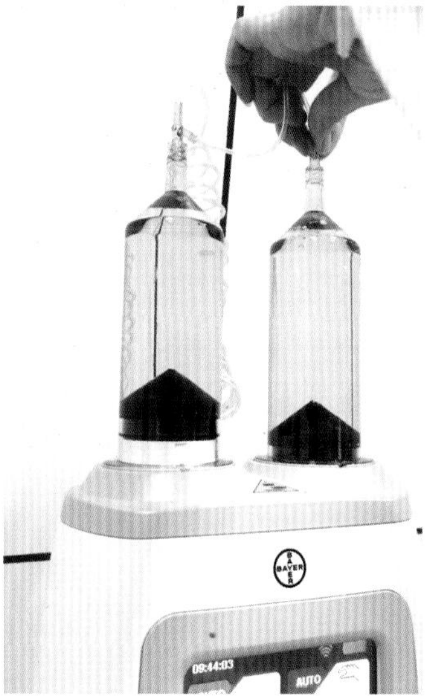

4.与留置针相连，注意不要进入气体。

Connect with the pin and be careful the gas doesn't enter.

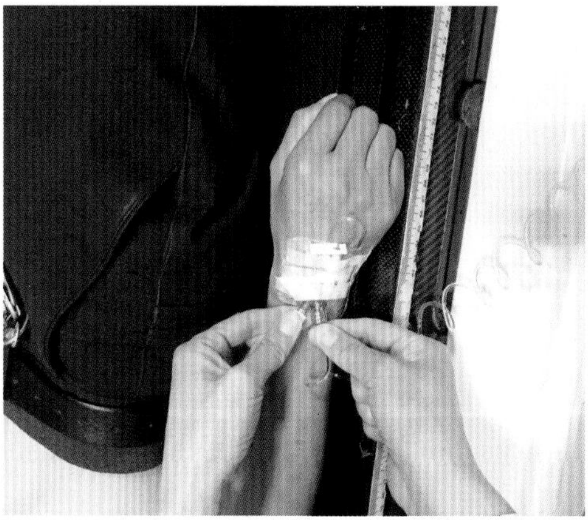

5. 设置流速、流量、压力等参数。

Set parameters such as flow quantity, velocity and pressure.

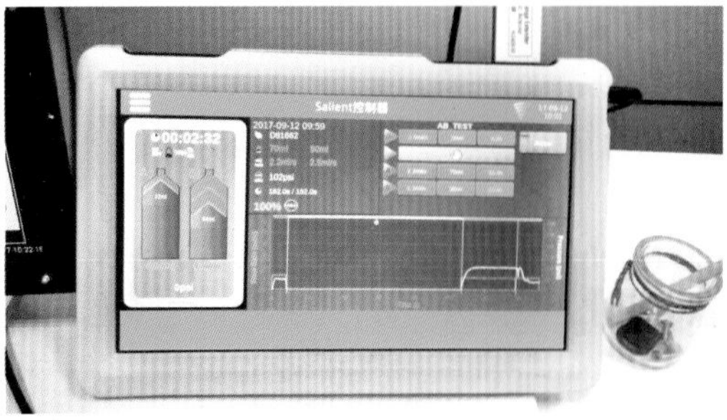

6. 在按动注射按钮前要再次确认输液管连接、注射参数设置情况。

Confirm that the infusion tube is connected, the injection parameters are set before press injection button.

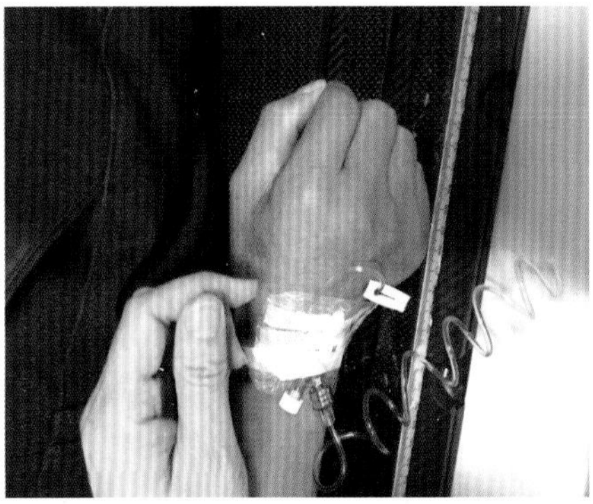

7. 注射过程中严密观察注射器工作状态及患者情况，出现异常状况停止注射。

During the injection, the injector and the patient was closely observed. If there is abnormal condition, stop injecting.

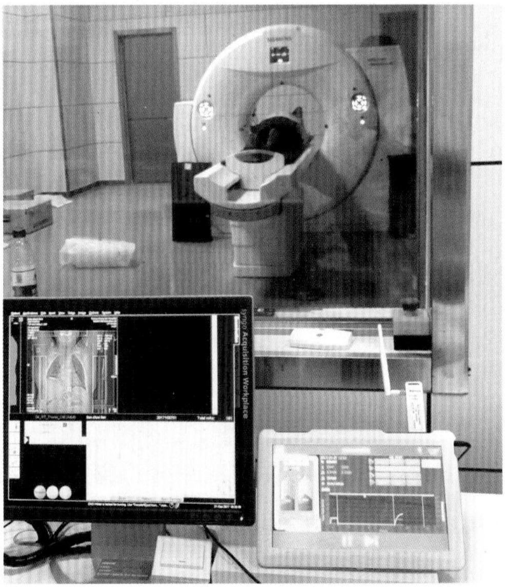

8.卸下针筒，关闭电源开关，清洁设备。

Unplug the needle, turn off the power, clean the equipment.

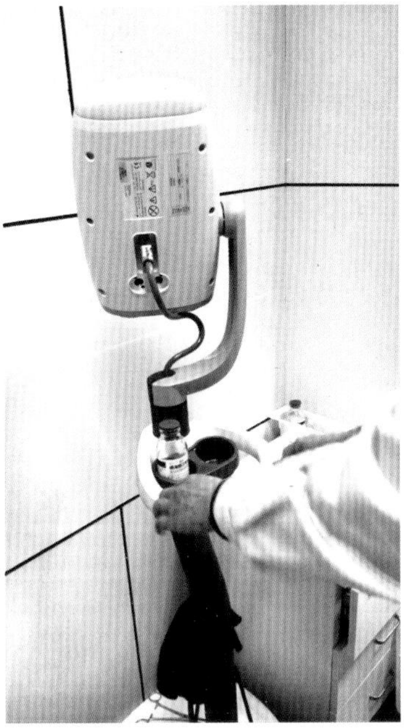

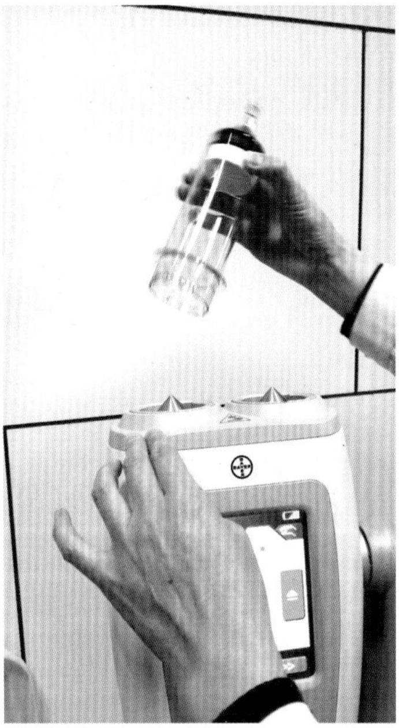

第29节　甘肃重离子医院重离子放射治疗楼辐射事故应急预案

Emergency Plan for Radiation Accidents in Heavy Ion Radiotherapy Buildings of Gansu Heavy Ion Hospital

为规范和强化应对突发重离子放射治疗楼辐射事故的应急处置能力，将重离子放射治疗楼辐射事故造成的损失和污染后果降低到最低程度，最大限度地保障放射工作人员与公众的安全，维护正常、和谐的放射诊疗秩序，做到重离子放射治疗楼辐射事故早发现、速报告、快处理，建立快速反应机制。按照上级环保部门、辐射安全部门与卫生行政部门要求，根据《职业病防治法》《放射诊疗管理规定》《辐射安全事故管理规定》《辐射安全事故应急处理预案》、国务院第449号令《放射性同位素与射线装置安全和防护条例》、卫生部《全国突发公共卫生事件应急预案》和卫生部第16号令《放射事故管理规定》等相关法律法规，特制定《甘肃重离子医院重离子治疗楼辐射事故应急预案》。

In order to standardize and strengthen the emergency response capacity to deal with radiation accidents in emergency heavy ion radiotherapy buildings, minimize the damage and pollution consequences caused by radiation accidents in heavy ion radiotherapy buildings, maximize the safety of radiation workers and the public, maintain normal and harmonious radiotherapy order, early detection, rapid reporting, and rapid processing of radiation accidents in heavy ion radiotherapy buildings should be implemented to establish a rapid response mechanism. In accordance with the requirements of the superior environmental protection department, radiation safety department and health administrative department, according to *Occupational Diseases Prevention and Control Law, Regulations on Radiological Diagnosis and Treatment, Regulations on the Administration of Radiation Safety Incidents, Precautions for Emergency Handling of Radiation Safety Accidents, Regulations on the Safety and Protection of Radioisotope and Radioactive Devices* of the State Council, Decree No. 449, and Ministry of Health *The national contingency plans for public health emergencies* and the 16th order of the Ministry of Health *Regulations on the Management of Radioactive Accidents* and other relevant laws and regulations, *Emergency Plan for Radiation Accidents in Heavy Ion Radiotherapy Buildings in Gansu Heavy Ion Hospital* is specially formulated.

1 组织机构及职责

(Organization and responsibilities)

我院参照武威市辐射事故应急指挥部的组织结构，成立重离子放射治疗楼辐射安全与防护领导小组、现场处置组、医疗救护组、设备抢修组、后勤协调组等，负责本院辐射事故（HIMM治疗终端误入、HIMM机房人员误入、HIMM机房通风系统故障等典型事故）应急处置调度和医疗救护工作。

According to the organizational structure of the radiation accident emergency command department of Wuwei City, our hospital establishes the Leading Group for Radiation Safety and Protection of Heavy Ion Radiotherapy Buildings, on-site disposal team, medical rescue team, equipment repair team, logistic coordination group, etc., which are responsible for emergency dispatching and medical rescue operations of the radiation accident at this hospital (typical accidents including HIMM treatment terminal accidental entry, misplacement of personnel in the HIMM room, failure of the ventilation system in the HIMM room, and so on).

1.1 领导小组（Leading group）

职业指导：辐射安全与防护领导小组，总体负责本院辐射安全与防护的规划和协调工作。具体工作包括：成立各专业小组，审核各小组成员的从业资质，建立健全辐射安全与防护应急队伍；至少配备一名注册核安全工程师担任常务副组长，处理本院辐射安全与防护的日常工作；建立并健全放射工作人员个人剂量档案和职业健康监护档案管理制度；其余成员为理工类专业或医学类专业背景的工作人员，负责对接和落实领导小组内本专业相关的具体工作；编制《辐射事故应急预案》，组织应急准备工作，调度人员，协调、落实和参加应急队伍的培训计划，每年至少组织一次辐射事故应急演练工作；对辐射事故发生后的应急行动进行组织协调、安排救助，总揽辐射事故应急救援行动；组织辐射安全与防护科普宣传，普及辐射安全基本知识和辐射事故预防常识，增强公众的自我防范意识和相关心理准备，提高公众防范辐射事故的能力，构建核安全文化；根据事故等级按规定时间向上级部门逐级报告；根据事故处理结果，解除安全警戒，负责恢复本单位正常秩序。

Career Guidance: The Radiation Safety and Protection Leading Group is responsible for the planning and coordination of radiation safety and protection in the hospital. Specific tasks include: Establish professional teams, review the qualifications of members of each team, establish a sound emergency radiation safety and protection team, and employ at least one registered nuclear safety engineer as an executive deputy leader to handle the daily work of radiation safety and protection in this hospital; establish and improve radiologists' personal dossier files and occupational health surveillance file management system; the remaining members are professionals from the science and engineering majors or have medical professional backgrounds; they are responsible for the docking and implementation of specific tasks related to this profession within the leading group; prepare *Radio accident emergency plan*, organize emergency preparedness, dispatch personnel, coordinate, implement and participate in the training plan of the emergency team, organize at least one radiation accident emergency drill per year; organize and coordinate emergency actions after radiation accidents, arrange assistance, and take responsibility for radiation accident emergency rescue operations; organize scientific propaganda on radiation safety and protection, popularize basic knowledge of radiation safety and prevention of radiation accidents, enhance public awareness of self-prevention and related psychological preparations, increase public ability to prevent radiation accidents, and build nuclear safety culture; according to the accident level report in the stipulated time level by level to the higher authorities; according to the results of incident handling, lift of security alert, be responsible for recovering the normal order of the unit.

在以下情况下可以解除安全警戒：

在安全连锁、防护装置经过维修工程人员的检修维护，能够有效发挥功能效用，工作场所和周围环境的辐射剂量经过现场处置专业技术人员检测，辐射剂量已降低至本底剂量水平，确认射线束、放射源得到有效控制的情况下，领导小组总负责人报上级环保、核与辐射及卫生行政部门批准后，可以解除安全警戒，恢复正常治疗秩序。

Security alert can be lifted under the following conditions:

When safety is interlocked, the protective device is overhauled and maintained by the maintenance engineer and can effectively function, the radiation dose at the workplace and surrounding environment is detected by professional technicians at the site, the radiation dose has been reduced to the background dose level, and the radiation beam and radioactive sources are effectively controlled, after the leading person in charge of the leading group reporting to the environmental protection, nuclear, radiation, and sanitation administrative departments at the next higher level for approval, the security alert can be lifted and the normal treatment order can be restored.

事故发生后的主要职责：

The main responsibilities after the accident:

（1）组织应急准备工作，调度人员，指挥现场工作。

Organize emergency preparedness, dispatch personnel, and direct on-site work.

（2）对重离子放射治疗楼辐射事故的现场进行组织协调、安排救助，指挥重离子放射治疗楼辐射事故应急救援行动。

Organize and coordinate the scene of radiation accidents in heavy ion radiotherapy buildings, arrange rescues, and direct emergency rescue operations for radiation accidents in heavy ion radiotherapy buildings.

（3）辐射安全与防护应急领导小组组长叶延程院长根据事故等级按规定时间向上级部门逐级报告。

Director Ye Yancheng, leader of the Emergency Leadership Team for Radiation Safety and Protection, reports to the higher authorities level by level in the stipulated time according to the level of the accident.

（4）恢复本单位正常秩序。

Restore the normal order of the unit.

应急办公室设置在重离子治疗楼一楼办公区。联系人：赵宏斌（13993558851）

The emergency office is located in the office area on the first floor of the heavy ion radiotherapy building. Person to contact: Zhao Hongbin （13993558851）

1.2 现场处置组（On-site disposal group）

辐射事故现场处置的成员由两部分组成：一为专业技术人员；二为安保警戒人员。

The members of the radiation accident site disposal consist of two parts, one is a professional technician and the other is a security guard.

职业指导：事故现场专业技术人员

Career guidance: Experts at the accident scene

具体落实辐射事故现场的处置工作，负有第一时间对发生、发现的辐射事故做出响应的职责，检测事故污染区，划定警戒区域，疏散事故现场其他人员，实施现场警戒，申请启动《辐射事故应急预案》。成员分别包括物理学、核技术等理工类、现场从事放射治疗的专业技术人员，对辐射安全与防护工作有常识性的认知，对辐射事故引起的伤害有足够高的意识，会使用、操作表面沾污仪、环境剂量监测仪、辐射剂量报警仪、放射性活度计，熟悉剂量监测系统和剂量监测报警系统，及时察觉环境剂量异常状况并上报领导小组。能够承担对事故现场进行现场污染水平监测和采样分析工作，划定受污染区域，做好应急现场的辐射防护工作；能够承担调查事故概况及所涉及的源项，分析事故原因、提出事故处置建议措施；能够承担监测和分析数据的整理和报告收集；能够根据现场调查结果并参考专家意见提出事故处置措施的建议；能够承担收集相关的法律、法规；承担事故分析和评价（包括事故分级和评价）及事故源项可能导致的剂量，预测和评价事故后果。参加各级环保、核与辐射安全部门的培训，提高核与辐射安全意识，积极参与构建核安全文化氛围。

Do the specific implementation of radiation accident site disposal work, have responsibility of responding to the occurrence and discovery of radiation accidents at the first time, detect accidental pollution areas, delineate alert areas, evacuate other personnel at the scene of the accident, do the implementation of on - site alert, apply to start the *Radiation Emergency*

Response Plan. Members are composed of physics, nuclear technology, and other professional and technical personnel who are engaged in radiation therapy. They have common - sense knowledge of radiation safety and protection work, and have a high awareness of the damage caused by radiation accidents, and can operate surface contamination meter, environmental dose monitor, radiation dose alarm meter, radioactivity meter, be familiar with dose monitoring system and dose monitoring alarm system, be timely aware of environmental dose abnormalities and report to the leading group. They can undertake on - site pollution level monitoring and sampling analysis work on the accident site, delineate the contaminated area, do a good job of radiation protection on the emergency site, be able to bear the investigation of the accident overview and the source of the involved items, analyze the cause of the accident, put forward the accident treatment proposal measures; can undertake monitoring and analysis of data collation and report collection; can make recommendations for accident treatment measures based on site survey results and with reference to expert advice; can afford to collect relevant laws and regulations; undertake accident analysis and evaluation (including accident classification and evaluation) of the doses that may be caused by the source of the accident, predict and evaluate the consequences of the accident. Participate in the training of environmental protection, nuclear and radiation safety departments at all levels, raise awareness of nuclear and radiation safety, and actively participate in building a nuclear safety culture atmosphere.

职业指导：事故现场安保警戒人员

Career guidance: Security guards at the scene of the accident

辐射事故现场的安保人员应具备执行治安保卫、安全警戒任务的经验，辐射事故发生后根据现场处置检测人员的检测结论、现场勘验情况，配合划定警戒线范围并进行现场警戒，组织事故现场的安全保卫、治安管理和交通疏导，维护现场秩序，保护事故现场；必要时通报或疏散周围单位和群众；协助营救受害人员，阻止无关人员随意靠近现场；协助有关部门采取必要的控制措施。

The security personnel at the scene of radiation accidents should have the experience of performing security and security alert tasks. After the occurrence of a radiation accident, according to the testing results of the on - site disposal and inspection personnel and on - site inspection conditions, the perimeter of the security line is coordinated and the alert is organized to organize the safeguarding, security management and traffic grooming of the sit of accident, maintain on - site order, protect accident scenes. Report or evacuate nearby units and people when necessary. Assist victims in the rescue, prevent unrelated persons from approaching the site at will, and assist relevant departments in taking necessary control measures.

现场检测、防护和通信设备：

On-site inspection, protection and communications equipment:

辐射巡测仪、α/β/γ表面污染监测仪、中子当量仪、个人剂量报警仪；铅衣、铅帽、铅围裙、铅手套、铅围脖、铅眼镜等；警示牌、警戒线、对讲机等。

Radiation tester, alpha/beta/gamma surface contamination monitor, neutron equivalence meter, personal dose alarm; lead clothing, lead lead, lead apron, lead gloves, lead collar, lead glasses, etc.; warning signs, cordon, Walkie-talkie and so on.

通过以下设备监测觉察放射线束泄漏或异常的状况：

The following devices are used to monitor the detection of radiation beam leakage or abnormal conditions:

安全连锁失效、防护装置失效、剂量监控设备失灵及操作者麻痹大意会导致放射线束泄漏，造成辐射事故。本院监测工作场所及周围环境辐射剂量变化的设备有：固定式环境剂量监测仪（NT6103A）、工作场所剂量监测报警系统（SB-1）、工作场所及环境辐射监测系统（伽马探测器：FHT191N，中子探测器：WEND3）。使用这一类定点放置的设备，可根据报警阈值定点监测和及时察觉放射线束泄漏，通报工作场所和周围环境辐射剂量异常的状况。除此之外，还可使用手持式、便携式、移动式环境剂量监测仪（FJ-347A）、个人剂量监测报警系统（FJ3500）、个人X/γ辐射剂量报警仪（BS2010）、表面沾污仪（RDS-80）、放射性活度计（CRC-25R）、放射性活度计（PM-905A）等设备，来检测工作场所和周围环境的辐射剂量状况。

Failure of the safety interlock, failure of the protective device, failure of the dose monitoring equipment, and operator incontinence can lead to radiation beam leakage and radiation accidents. The hospital's equipments for monitoring changes in radiation dose at the workplace and in the surrounding environment include: fixed environmental dose monitor (NT6103A), workplace dose monitoring system (SB-1), workplace and environmental radiation monitoring system (gamma detectors: FHT191N, neutron detector: WEND3). Using this type of fixed-point placement device, monitoring based on alarm thresholds and timely detection of radiation beam leaks can be used to notify the workplace and surrounding environment of radiation dose abnormalities. In addition, hand-held, portable, mobile environmental dose monitor (FJ-347A), personal dose monitoring alarm system (FJ3500), personal X/gamma radiation dose alarm (BS2010), and surface contaminants (RDS-80), radioactivity meter (CRC-25R), radioactivity meter (PM-905A) and other equipment can be used to detect the radiation dose status of the workplace and the surrounding environment.

事故发生后的主要职责：

The main responsibilities after the accident:

（1）治疗大厅现场操作人员（放疗技师）是辐射事故的发现人，发现HIMM治疗终端误入、HIMM机房人员误入或HIMM机房通风故障等事故时，立即通知（对讲机呼叫）中控室关闭束流闸、停止供束，同时向现场处置组负责人祁央（13993503180）报告，请求支援。

The on - site operator (radiotherapy technician) of the treatment hall is the discoverer of the radiation accident and immediately notices (interphone call) the central control room to close beam flow gate, stop the beam, when the terminal of HIMM treatment is mistakenly entered, the personnel of the HIMM room is mistakenly entered, or the ventilation of the HIMM room is faulty at the same time, report to the head of the on - site disposal group Qi Ying (13993503180), request support.

（2）现场处置组负责人祁英接到重离子放射治疗楼辐射事故发生的报告后，立即带领现场处置组成员携带检测和防护设备赶赴现场，首先采取措施保护工作人员和公众的生命安全，保护环境不受污染，最大限度地控制事态发展，同时向辐射安全与领导小组负责人叶延程院长汇报，申请全面启动辐射事故应急预案。

After receiving a report on the occurrence of a radiation accident in a heavy ion radiotherapy building, Qi Ying, the person in charge of the on - site disposal group, immediately led the on - site disposal team members to bring testing and protective equipment to the scene. First, they take measures to protect the safety of workers and the public, and to protect the environment not to be polluted and the developments are controlled to the maximum extent. At the same time, they report to Dean Ye Yancheng, head of the Radiation Safety and Leading Group, and apply for full launch of emergency plans for radiation accidents.

（3）专业技术人员使用剂量报警设备勘验、划定紧急隔离区，安保人员负责现场警戒，禁止无关人员进入，保护好现场。

The professional and technical personnel use the dose alarm equipment to inspect and delineate the emergency isolation zone. The security personnel are responsible for on - the - spot alerting and prohibit the entry of unrelated personnel to protect the site.

（4）专业人员迅速、正确判断事件性质，将事故情况报告重离子放射治疗楼辐射事故应急工作领导小组组长叶延程院长。

Professionals quickly and correctly judge the nature of the incident and report the accident to Dean Ye Yancheng, leader of the Leading Group for Radiation Accidents Emergency Treatment at the Heavy Ion Radiotherapy Building.

（5）配合上级卫生行政主管部门对事故进行立案调查、检测和现场处理等各项工作。

Cooperate with superior health administrative department to carry out various tasks such as investigation of the accident, detection and on - site treatment.

1.3 医疗救护组（Medical care team）

职业指导：辐射事故医疗救护

Career Guidance: Radiation accident medical care

辐射事故医疗救护组，遵照辐射安全与防护领导小组命令，具体落实辐射事故现场医疗救护工作。成员包括专业放疗医师和护士，有必要的辐射损伤处理和紧急救护经验。按照辐射事故救护原则及措施实施医学救护、辐射事故现场伤员的抢救，遵循分级救治并坚持先重后轻和快抢、快救、快送的原则，尽快将伤员撤离核辐射事故现场。根据其损伤程度和各期不同的特点及实际条件，积极采用中西医结合综合救治措施，使之得到及时、有效、合理的救治。

The Radiation Accident Medical Care Team, in compliance with the order of the Leading Group on Radiation Safety and Protection, specifically implements the medical rescue work at the radiation accident site. The members are composed of professional radiotherapy physicians and nurses, and have the necessary radiation damage management and emergency care experience. According to the radiation accident rescue principles and measures to implement medical rescue, the rescue of the wounded on the scene of the radiation accident, follow the principle of grading treatment and adhere to the first heavy light and fast rob, fast rescue, fast delivery, remove the injured from the nuclear radiation accident site as soon as possible. According to the degree of injury and the different characteristics and actual conditions of each period, actively adopt treatment measures of integrated traditional Chinese and western medicine so as to obtain timely, effective and reasonable treatment.

医学应急装备：

Medical emergency equipment:

外科器械、输血装置、血细胞计数器、显微镜、制造血液图片设备、收集储藏生物样品的容器、穿刺箱、救护面罩、除颤仪、急救箱、急救药品、抗生素、局部使用药膏、取样设备、氧气袋、消毒用品、平车等。

Surgical instruments, blood transfusion devices, blood cell counters, microscopes, equipment for making blood pictures, containers for storing biological samples, penetrating boxes, rescue masks, defibrillators, first aid kits, emergency medicines, antibiotics, topical ointments, sampling equipment, oxygen bags , disinfection supplies, flat cars and so on.

事故发生后的主要职责：

The main responsibilities after the accident:

（1）接到领导小组命令后，带领医疗救护组人员，携带急救药品、器具等医学应急装备迅速赶赴现场。

After receiving the order of the leading group, the medical rescue team should carry emergency medical supplies and equipment and other medical emergency equipment to the scene.

（2）现场进行伤员救助，并根据现场情况向领导小组报告人员损伤情况，联系相关科室，跟随救治。

Rescue the wounded on the scene, and report the injury situation to the leading group according to the situation on the site, contact relevant departments, and follow the treatment.

（3）通知后勤保障组提供车辆和应急物资，如发生Ⅲ级以上辐射事故，立即联系甘肃省辐射救治基地（甘肃省人民医院），运送和陪护本院无法救治的事故伤患到基地进一步救治。

Inform the Logistic Support Group to provide vehicles and emergency supplies. If a radiation accident of class Ⅲ or higher occurs, contact the Gansu Provincial Radiation Treatment Base（People' s Hospital of Gansu Province）immediately to transport and escort the accidental patients who cannot be treated in this hospital to further treatment at the base.

（4）将人员恢复情况随时上报应急领导小组。

The personnel recovery situation will be reported to the emergency leadership team at any time.

辐射事故发生后，救护人员可采取的医疗措施如下：

After the radiation accident, the medical measures that the ambulance personnel can be taken are as follows:

①现场救治

根据受照人员的初期症状和外周血淋巴细胞绝对数等迅速估计伤情。伤员受照剂量小于0.1Gy者只作一般医学检查；受照剂量大于0.25Gy者应予对症治疗；受照剂量大于0.5Gy应住院观察，并予及时治疗；受照剂量大于1Gy者，必须住院严密观察和治疗。中度以上放射损伤者应尽早口服抗放药523片30 mg，有初期反应者应及时给予对症处理。外照射急性放射病病人，根据GB8281—1997《外照射急性放射病的诊断标准及处理原则》采取综合性治疗。除了受核辐射损伤外，如果伤员还合并有冲击伤、烧伤等损伤，则应同时按照冲击伤、烧伤等相应的处理方法进行自救互救。

On-site treatment

According to the initial symptoms of the affected person and the absolute number of peripheral blood lymphocytes, etc., the injury is quickly estimated. If the dose is less than 0.1 Gy, only the general medical examination is required; if the dose is greater than 0.25 Gy, the wounded should be treated symptomatically; if the dose is greater than 0.5 Gy, the wounded should be observed in hospital and promptly treated; if the dose is greater than 1 Gy, the wounded must be hospitalized, and take close observation and treatment. Patients with moderate or above radiation injury should take oral anti-radiation drug 523 tablets 30 mg as soon as possible, and initial response should be given to symptomatic treatment in time. For patients with acute radiation sickness after external exposure, comprehensive treatment shall be taken according to GB8281-1997 *Diagnostic criteria and principles of treatment of acute radiation sickness from external radiation*. In addition to injuries caused by nuclear radiation, if the injured person also incorporates injuries such as impact injuries and burns, he or she should be rescued and rescues each other according to the corresponding treatment methods such as impact injuries and burns.

②早期治疗

早期治疗由辐射事故地区附近的早期治疗机构组织实施。伤员体表放射性沾染超过控制水平者，应进行全身洗消。食入放射性物质者，在口服碘化钾片的基础上，应及时进行催吐或洗胃等。漏服抗放药523片、碘化钾片的伤员，应及时补服；因严重呕吐不能口服523片的伤员，应及早肌肉注射抗放药500一次，10mg。初步诊断为中度以上急性放射病者，在应用523或500的基础上，再口服抗放药408片300 mg，并给予对症处理。重度以上急性放射病伤员，静脉滴注低分子右旋糖酐，伤情偏重者，预防性使用抗生素等药物。早期治疗机构留治轻度骨髓型急性放射病和不宜后送的放射病伤员。

Early treatment

Early treatment is organized by early treatment institutions near the radiation accident area. The injured person whose body surface has been irradiated more than the control level by radioactive contamination should undergo general decontamination. In case of ingestion of radioactive material, vomiting or gastric lavage should be promptly performed besides orally taking potassium iodide tablets. Patients who missed the anti-radiation drug 523 tablets and potassium iodide tablets should be given promptly to take the service; due to severe vomiting, patients who cannot orally take 523 tablets, should be injected intramuscularly anti-radiation drug 500, 10 mg once. Patients with a primary diagnosis of acute radiation sickness above moderate level should be given anti-radiation drug 408 tablets 300 mg orally besides the application of 523 or 500, and given symptomatic treatment. Severe acute radiation sickness wounded, intravenous infusion of low-molecular dextran should be taken. If the injury situation is heavier, prophylacticly use antibiotics and other drugs. The early treatment institutions should hold patients who have been diagnosed mild bone marrow-type acute radiation sickness and radiation sickness wounded who should not be evacuated.

③专科治疗

急性放射病专科治疗，通常由专科医院或综合性医院相应的专科来组织实施。

Specialist treatment

Specialized treatment for acute radiation sickness is usually organized by the corresponding specialties of a specialist hospital or a general hospital.

1.4 设备抢修组（Equipment repair team）

职业指导：辐射事故设备抢修

辐射事故的设备抢修人员是电气设备维修专业背景的专业技术人员，具有设备故障检查、故障维修和排除的职业素养，熟悉造成安全连锁失灵、失效的可能原因，可熟练使用维修工具检查设备故障，查明事故原因，维修现场故障设备，为恢复正常工作状态提供设备维修维护的保障。同时对辐射安全与防护的知识有一定程度的了解和学习，与辐射事故现场处置人员保持沟通，进入事故现场时懂得采取必要的防护措施。

Career guidance: Radiation accident equipment repair

The equipment repair personnel for radiation accidents are professional technicians in the professional background of electrical equipment maintenance. They have professional qualifications for equipment failure inspection, fault repair, and troubleshooting. They are familiar with the possible causes of safety interlock failures and failures, and can be proficient in using maintenance tools to inspect equipment, faults, identify the cause of the accident, and repair the faulty equipment on site, and provide equipment maintenance and maintenance guarantees for restoring normal working conditions. At the same time, they have a certain degree of understanding and learning about the radiation safety and protection knowledge, and maintain communication with the radiation accident site disposal personnel and know how to take necessary protective measures when entering the accident site.

事故发生后的主要职责：

The main responsibilities after the accident:

（1）接到领导小组命令后，立即带领维修人员携带维修工具赶赴现场检查设备故障，抢修设备；

After receiving the order of the leading group, immediately lead the maintenance personnel to bring the maintenance tools to the site to check the equipment failure and repair the equipment.

（2）查明事故原因，维修现场故障设备，并做好记录，向领导小组汇报。

Identify the cause of the accident, repair the on-site fault equipment, and make a record, report to the leading group.

1.5 后勤保障组（Logistics support group）

职业指导：应急响应后勤保障

应急响应后勤保障人员应该熟悉应急人员、设施和应急物资的保障工作，在辐射事故发生时保证水、电、通讯和应急物资供应，派遣车辆等交通运输工具，保证食物用餐和饮水。

Career guidance: Emergency response logistics support

Emergency response logistics support personnel should be familiar with emergency personnel, facilities, and emergency supplies. They should ensure the supply of water, electricity, communications, and emergency supplies in the event of a radiation accident, and dispatch vehicles and other transportation vehicles to ensure food meals and drinking water is served.

事故发生后的主要职责：

The main responsibilities after the accident:

（1）接到领导小组命令后，立即启动应急设施和发放应急物资；

Immediately after receiving the order of the leading group, emergency facilities and emergency supplies were started.

（2）保证水、电、通讯和应急物资供应，派遣车辆等交通运输工具；

Ensure the supply of water, electricity, communications and emergency supplies, and dispatch vehicles and other means of transport.

（3）保证食物用餐和饮水；

Ensure food meals and drinking water.

（4）记录应急物资、食物饮水发放情况和车辆派遣情况，向领导小组汇报。

Record emergency supplies, distribution of food and drinking water, and dispatch of vehicles, and report to the leading group.

2 典型辐射事故应急措施

（Measures for typical radiation accident emergency）

2.1 HIMM治疗终端误入

HIMM treatment terminal entered incorrectly

2.1.1 事故设定

Accident settings

我院重离子加速器HIMM治疗终端在做治疗时，突然发生分区管理失效、安全连锁装置失效或工作人员误操作等导致人员误入治疗终端。我院工作人员立即用对讲机呼叫通知中控室切断束流、积极采取相应措施及立即疏散撤离辐射区范围的人员。HIMM治疗终端误入事故应急工作领导小组火速组织相关人员进行事故处理，并进行事后调查、分析、总结。

During the treatment of the HIMM heavy ion accelerator treatment terminal in our hospital, the zone management or the safety interlock are out of control suddenly, or wrong operation caused some person entered the treatment terminal incorrectly. The staff of our hospital immediately inform the central control room with the intercom call to cut off the beam, take emergency measures and immediately evacuate the personnel out of radioactive area. The leading team of the HIMM treatment terminal accidental organize deal with accidents immediately and make investigate, analysis and summery after the event.

2.1.2 可能原因分析

Analyze the possible reason

①分区管理失效；

The zone management out of control.

②安全连锁装置失效；

The safety interlock system invalid.

③工作人员误操作。

Wrong operation from staff.

2.1.3 此类辐射事故应急措施

Emergency measures for such radiation accidents

①立即停止出束；

Stop the beam immediately.

②启动辐射事故应急预案；

Start emergency plan for radiation accidents.

③画出警戒线，疏散非事故处理人员；

Set cordon, evacuate unrelated personnel.

④进行现场辐射环境监测；

Measure environment radiation on-site.

⑤对受误照射人员进行生命体征检查，采取医疗救治措施。

Inspect vital signs on exposed personnel and take rescue measures.

2.1.4 此类辐射事故主要预防措施

Major preventive measures for such radiation accidents

①加强分区管理和巡察力度；

Strengthen zone management and inspection efforts.

②定期对安全连锁的有效性进行检查；

Regularly check the effectiveness of safety interlock.

③加强工作人员的技能培训与考核；

Strengthen staff skills training and assessment.

④严格按照安全操作规程进行操作。

Strictly follow safe operating procedures.

2.2 HIMM机房人员误入事故

HIMM treatment room entered incorrectly

2.2.1 事故设定

Accident settings

我院重离子加速器HIMM机房在做治疗时，突然发生分区管理失效、安全连锁装置失效或工作人员误操作等导致人员误入。我院工作人员立即用对讲机呼叫通知中控室切断束流、积极采取相应措施及对辐射区范围的病人立即疏散撤离。HIMM机房人员误入事故应急工作领导小组火速组织相关人员进行事故处理，并进行事后调查、分析、总结。

During the treatment of the HIMM heavy ion accelerator treatment room in our hospital, the zone management or the safety interlock out of control suddenly, or wrong operation caused some person stray into the treatment room. The staff of our hospital immediately informed the central control room with the intercom call to cut off the beam, take emergency measures and immediately evacuate the personnel out of radioactive area . The leading team of the HIMM treatment room entered incorrectly accidental organize deal with accidents immediately and make investigate, analysis and summery after the event.

2.2.2 可能原因分析

Analyze the possible reason

①分区管理失效；

The zone management out of control.

②安全连锁装置失效；

The safety interlock system invalid.

③工作人员误操作。

Wrong operation from staff.

2.2.3 此类辐射事故应急措施

Emergency measures for such radiation accidents

①立即停止出束；

Stop the beam immediately.

②启动辐射事故应急预案；

Start emergency plan for radiation accidents.

③划出警戒线，疏散非事故处理人员；

Set cordon, evacuation unrelated personnel.

④进行现场辐射环境监测；

Measure environment radiation on-site.

⑤对受误照射人员进行生命体征检查，采取医疗救治措施。

Inspect vital signs on exposed personnel and take rescue measures.

2.2.4　此类辐射事故主要预防措施

Major preventive measures for such radiation accidents

①加强分区管理和巡察力度；

Strengthen zone management and inspection efforts.

②定期对安全连锁的有效性进行检查；

Regularly check the effectiveness of safety interlock.

③加强工作人员的技能培训与考核；

Strengthen staff skills training and assessment.

④严格按照安全操作规程进行操作。

Strictly follow safe operating procedures.

2.3　HIMM机房通风系统故障

（HIMM treatment room ventilation system malfunction）

2.3.1　事件设定

Accident settings

我院重离子加速器HIMM机房在做治疗时，突然发生断电、风机故障、人员误操作等导致通风系统故障。我院工作人员立即用对讲机呼叫通知中控室切断束流、积极采取相应措施及对治疗大厅内的人员立即疏散撤离。辐射事故应急工作领导小组火速组织相关人员进行事故处理，并进行事后调查、分析、总结。

During the treatment of the HIMM heavy ion accelerator treatment room in our hospital, power off, fan failure or staff take wrong operation cause ventilation system has malfunction. The staff of our hospital immediately informed the central control room with the intercom call to cut off the beam, take emergency measures and immediately evacuate the personnel out of radioactive area. The leading team of the emergency radiation accident organize deal with accidents immediately and make investigate, analysis and summery after the event.

2.3.2　可能原因分析

Analyze the possible reason

①断电；

Power off.

②风机故障；

The fan has malfunction.

③人员误操作造成停机。

Staff take wrong operation cause the fan stop working.

2.3.3 此类辐射事故应急措施

Emergency measures for such radiation accidents

①立即停止出束，对通风系统进行检查、维修；

Stop the beam immediately, check and repair the ventilation system.

②检查风机，若发生故障，立即维修或更换。

Inspect the fan and repair or replace it immediately if it fails.

2.3.4 此类辐射事故主要预防措施

Major preventive measures for such radiation accidents

①加强检查和监测；

Strengthen inspection and monitoring.

②定期对风机进行检查；

Check the fan regularly.

③设置备用风机和备用电源；

Prepare standby fan and standby power.

④加强管理和培训。

Strengthen management and training.

3 事件总结

(Accident summary)

本院辐射安全事故应急处置结束后，现场处置组、医疗救护组、设备抢修组、后勤保障组成员分别以书面形式向本组负责人汇报应急处置工作的结果和情况，各组负责人将情况汇总后向总负责人叶延程院长汇报。总负责人从辐射安全与防护领导小组中抽调人员组成调查小组，对事故原因进行调查，召集各组成员开会总结经验教训，以杜绝类似事故再次发生，做好相关记录，并将调查结果向上级部门汇报。

After the radiation safety accident disposition, each group need to report the results and circumstances of accident to the group leader in written form. And each group leader need to report to the general superintendent president Ye Yancheng. General superintendent need to investigate each team member to form a survey team. The survey team will investigate the causes of the accident. The members of each group will be called to meet and sum up experiences to prevent the similar accidents, make relevant records, and report the investigation results to the higher authorities.

参考文献

1. Shi D, Zhao X, Ning W, et al. Construction of hospital management information system from the perspective of patients[J]. China Market, 2018(32): 189-190.

师东菊，赵兴艳，宁伟东，等. 患方视角下的医院管理信息系统的构建［J］. 中国市场，2018（32）：189-190.

2. Meng X. Research on hospital information system construction in medical informatization[J]. China Health Industry, 2016(35): 66-67.

孟勋. 医疗信息化中的医院信息系统建设研究［J］. 中国卫生产业，2016（35）：66-67.

3.Lin F, Zeng Z, Wang Y . Discussing accuracy of radiotherapy for tumors[J]. Chinese Journal of Radiological Health, 2012(3): 310-311.

林锋，曾自力，王勇兵. 肿瘤放射治疗准确性的探讨［J］. 中国辐射卫生，2012（3）：310-311.

4.Fang F. Comparison of different body position fixation techniques in radiotherapy for thoracic and abdominal tumors[J]. Journal of Imaging Research and Medical Applications, 2018(21): 102-103.

方芳. 不同体位固定技术在胸腹部肿瘤放射治疗中的应用比较［J］. 影像研究与医学应用，2018（21）：102-103.

5. Wu B, Duan F. Application of Mask Fixing Technology in the Radiotherapy for Head and Neck Cancer[J]. Chinese Medical Equipment, 2007, 22(12): 96-98.

吴冰，段峰. 面罩固定技术在头颈部肿瘤放疗中的应用［J］. 中国医学装备，2007，22（12）：96-98.

6. 胡逸民，杨定宇. 肿瘤放射治疗技术［M］. 北京：北京医科大学中国协和医科大学联合出版社，1999.

7. 黄拔群，扬石山，柳耿淳，等. 改进头颈部恶性肿瘤外照射放疗技术的临床观察［J］. 中国医师杂志，2003（7）：916-918.

8.梁俊武，萧达宜.面罩固定在鼻咽癌照射野中的重复性及其方法的改进［J］.癌症，1999，18（增刊）：150-151.

9.范乃斌，夏廷毅，孙庆选，等.面罩固定不同标记法在重复摆位中的精度比较［J］.中华放射肿瘤学杂志，2009，9（3）：215-216.

10.Herman M G. Clinical use of electronic portal imaging［J］. Semin Radiat Oncol，2005,15: 157-167.

11.成尚利，何俊民.医学图像融合配准技术［J］.上海生物医学工程，2007，28（3）：171-175.

12.韩俊庆，王力军.放射治疗技术［M］.2版.北京：人民卫生出版社，2013.

13.胡逸民，杨定宇.肿瘤放射治疗技术［M］.北京：北京医学大学中国协和医科大学联合出版社，1999.

14.刘世耀.质子治疗设备的现状和发展［J］.基础医学和临床，2005（2）：123-125.

15.中华医学会重症医学分会.中国重症患者转运指南（2010）（草案)［J］.中国危重病急救医学，2010（22）：328-330.

16.林涵真，危丽华，董馨.急诊危重患者的院内转运体会［J］.中国误诊学杂志，2007，17（7）：4027.

17.胡逸民.放射治疗过程及其对剂量准确性的影响［M］//殷蔚伯，余子豪，徐国镇，等.肿瘤放射治疗学.4版.北京：中国协和医科大学出版社，2008：207-209.

18.胡逸民.治疗体位及体位固定技术［M］// 殷蔚伯，余子豪，徐国镇，等.肿瘤放射治疗学.4版.北京：中国协和医科大学出版社，2008：95-99.

19.王永成， 邓国忠.胸部肿瘤患者体位固定方法比较［J］.临床论坛， 2013，（1）：1-3.

20.白兰兰，田焕茹，姚婷.胸部肿瘤三维适形放疗摆位的重复性研究［J］.现代肿瘤医学， 2010，1（9）：2-3.

21.陈德路.胸腹部肿瘤放射治疗定位和摆位的研究与改进［J］.中国医学物理学杂志， 2010， 27（4）：2-3.

22.孙新臣， 孙向东， 马建新.肿瘤放射治疗技术学［M］.南京：东南大学出版社， 2015.

23.胡逸民，张红志，戴建荣.放射治疗的质量保证［M］//胡逸民.肿瘤放射物理学.北京：原子能出版社，1999：616.

24.江波，戴建荣.锥形束CT成像技术及其在放疗中的应用［J］.中华放射肿瘤学杂志，2010（3）：158-161.

25.殷蔚伯，余子豪，徐国镇，等.肿瘤放射治疗学［M］.4版.北京：中国协和医科大学出版社，2008.

26.高剑波.CT明医解读［M］.郑州：河南科学技术出版社，2013.

27.王书轩.CT读片指南［M］.2版.北京：化学工业出版社，2013.

28.刘新国，李强，杜晓刚，等.初步的IMP重离子治疗计划系统［J］.原子核物理评论，2010，27（4）：480-487.